Mind Maps
in Medicine

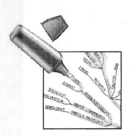

For Churchill Livingstone:

Publisher: Laurence Hunter
Project Editor: Janice Urquhart
Design and typesetting: Martin Coventry
Project Controller: Kay Hunston

Mind Maps® in Medicine

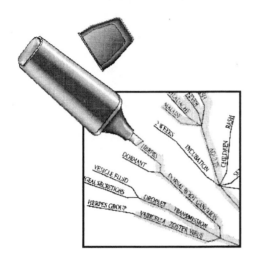

P. McDermott MB ChB FRCR
Consultant Radiologist,
Stirling Royal Infirmary NHS Trust, Stirling, UK

D.N. Clarke MB ChB FRCP
Consultant Physician,
Stirling Royal Infirmary NHS Trust, Stirling, UK

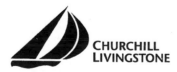
CHURCHILL
LIVINGSTONE

EDINBURGH LONDON NEW YORK OXFORD PHILADELPHIA ST LOUIS SYDNEY TORONTO 1998

CHURCHILL LIVINGSTONE
An imprint of Elsevier Limited

First published 1998
  Reprinted 1999
  Reprinted 2002
  Reprinted 2003, 2004

ISBN 0 443 05195 X

British Library of Cataloguing in Publication Data
A catalogue record for this book is available from the British
Library.

1004 913 136

Library of Congress Cataloging in Publication Data
A catalog record for this book is available from the Library of
Congress.

Mind Map is the Registered Trade Mark of the Buzam Organisation,
used with permission.

Medical knowledge is constantly changing. As new information
becomes available, changes in treatment, procedures, equipment and
the use of drugs become necessary. The authors and the publishers
have, as far as it is possible, taken care to ensure that the information
given in this text is accurate and up to date. However, readers are
strongly advised to confirm that the information, especially with
regard to drug usage, complies with current legislation and standards
of practice.

 ELSEVIER your source for books,
journals and multimedia
in the health sciences
www.elsevierhealth.com

Printed and bound by Antony Rowe Ltd, Eastbourne
Transferred to digital printing 2005

The
publisher's
policy is to use
paper manufactured
from sustainable forests

Preface

Mind Mapping, invented by Tony Buzan, results in increased confidence, saves precious studying time and gives the student a sense of achievement.

Conventional textbooks present information in such a way that the **key words** are not always obvious to the student. Research shows that **key words** are important in learning as they create and reinforce learning pathways.

The **key words** in this book are presented in the context of pathways which connect to form maps of each topic. The information on each topic is thus connected to provide a framework for revision and learning.

Studies show that revision of **key words** creates and strengthens word associations and helps the brain to process further information on the topic faster. Psychologists call this effect the 'semantic prime'.

The Mind Maps provide an overview of the subjects and are designed to 'prime' the brain to remember the information.

P.McD.
D.N.C.   Stirling 1997

Contents

How to use this Book

1. Always use a visual aid to move over the Mind Map — a marker, felt-tip pen, or even a finger and start at the 1 o'clock position on the Mind Map, moving clockwise. The more common features are mentioned first.

2. Work for about 25 minutes followed by a five minute break. Do not study for more than two hours at a time.

3. Quickly read over the topic in your textbook several times. Underline or highlight key words — remember this is your own book!

4. Minutes after the end of your study period turn to the relevant Mind Map. Use your highlighter or coloured pen to link or isolate groups of words on the map. Insert cross references to other maps and add any other points you wish to remember.

5. Revise the Mind Map the next day for a few minutes. Test yourself to see how much you have remembered.

6. Revise the Mind Maps fairly frequently emphasizing points made in lectures or tutorials. Continue to add to the map if you wish.

7. Revision of the Mind Maps just before going to bed can be useful — there is a theory that the brain consolidates information as you sleep.

Glossary of abbreviations

Ab	antibody
Abs	antibodies
ACA	anterior communicating artery
ACTH	adrenocorticotrophic hormone
AD	autosomal dominant
AF	atrial fibrillation
AIDS	acquired immunosuppressive disorder
ALK PHOS	alkaline phosphatase
AR	autosomal recessive
ARF	acute renal failure
ASD	atrial septal defect
BP	blood pressure
CD	collecting duct
CHD	congenital heart disease
CMV	cytomegalovirus
CNS	central nervous system
CPK	creatine phosphokinase
CRF	chronic renal failure
CRP	C reactive protein
CS	cavernous sinus
CSF	cerebrospinal fluid
CT	computed tomography
CXR	chest X-ray
DCT	distal convoluted tubule
DIC	disseminated intravascular coagulation
DVT	deep vein thrombosis
ECG	electrocardiograph
EEG	electroencephalograph
EM	electron micrograph
ERCP	endoscopic retrograde cholangio-pancreatography
ESP	especially
ESR	erythrocyte sedimentation rate
GBM	glomerular basement membrane
GFR	glomerular filtration rate
GIT	gastrointestinal tract
GM	gram stain
GN	glomerulonephritis
GUT	genitourinary tract
GVH	graft vs host disease
Hb	haemoglobin

HIV	human immunodeficiency virus		PTH	parathyroid hormone
ICA	internal carotid artery		PUO	pyrexia of unknown origin
ICP	intracranial pressure		RA	rheumatoid arthritis
Ig	immunoglobulin		RBC	red blood cell
IHD	ischaemic heart disease		RF	rheumatic fever
IM	intramuscular		RHD	rheumatic heart disease
INR	international normalised ratio		RV	right ventricle
IV	intravenous		RVF	right ventricular failure
IVC	inferior vena cava		RVH	right ventricular hypertrophy
JVP	jugular venous pressure		SAH	subarachnoid haemorrhage
LMN	lower motor neurone		SDH	subdural haemorrhage
LSE	left sternal edge		SLE	systemic lupus erythematosus
LUSE	left upper sternal edge		SS	systemic sclerosis (scleroderma)
LV	left ventricle		STAPH	staphylococcus
LVF	left ventricular failure		STREP	streptococcus
LVH	left ventricular hypertrophy		SUP	superior
MCA	middle cerebral artery		SY	syndrome (also Sy)
MI	myocardial infarction		TB	tuberculosis
MRI	magnetic resonance imaging		TIPS	transjugular intrahepatic portosystemic shunt
MS	multiple sclerosis		TSH	thyroid stimulating hormone
Nv	nerve		UMN	upper motor neurone
PCA	posterior communicating artery		US	ultrasound
PCT	proximal convoluted tubule		UTI	urinary tract infection
PCV	packed cell volume		VIP	very important piece
PDA	patent duct arteriosus		VIT	vitamin
PFTs	pulmonary function tests		VSD	ventricular septal defect
PN	polyarteritis nodosa		WBC	white blood cell
PTC	percutaneous transhepatic cholangiography		WT	weight

Cardiology

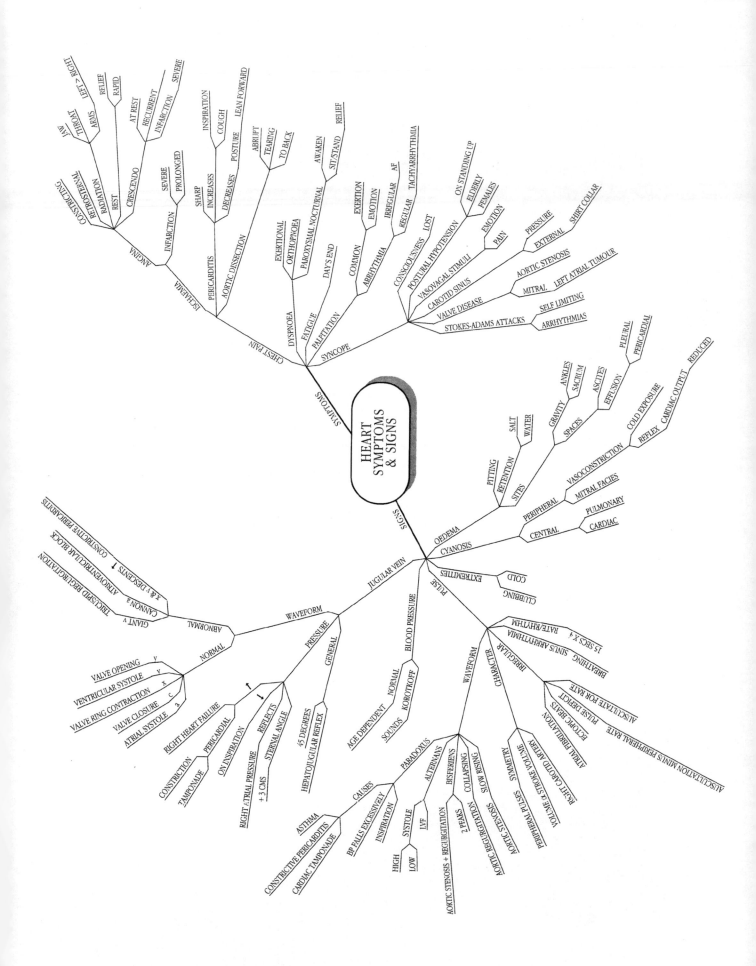

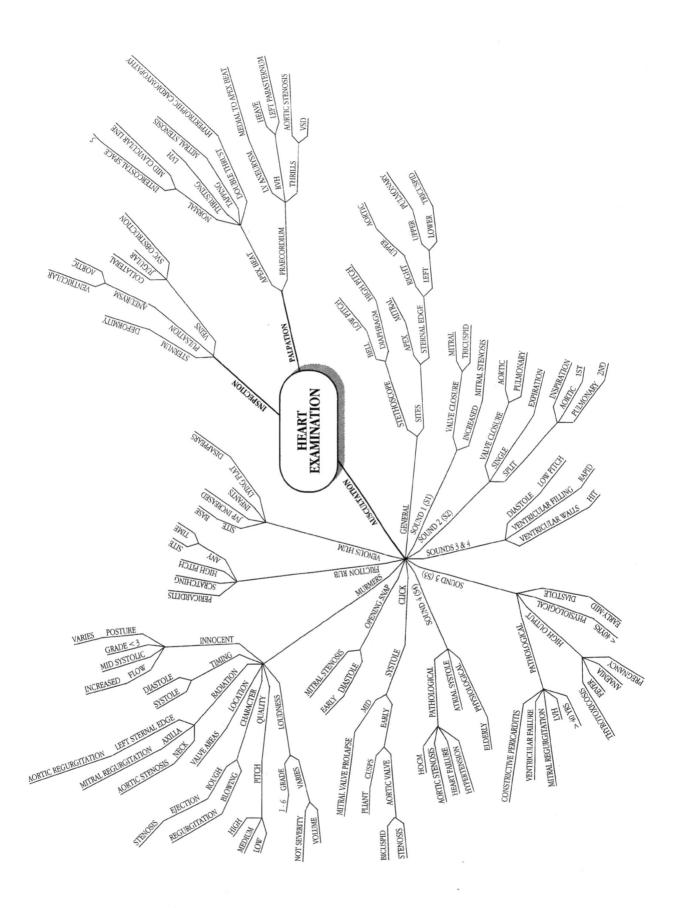

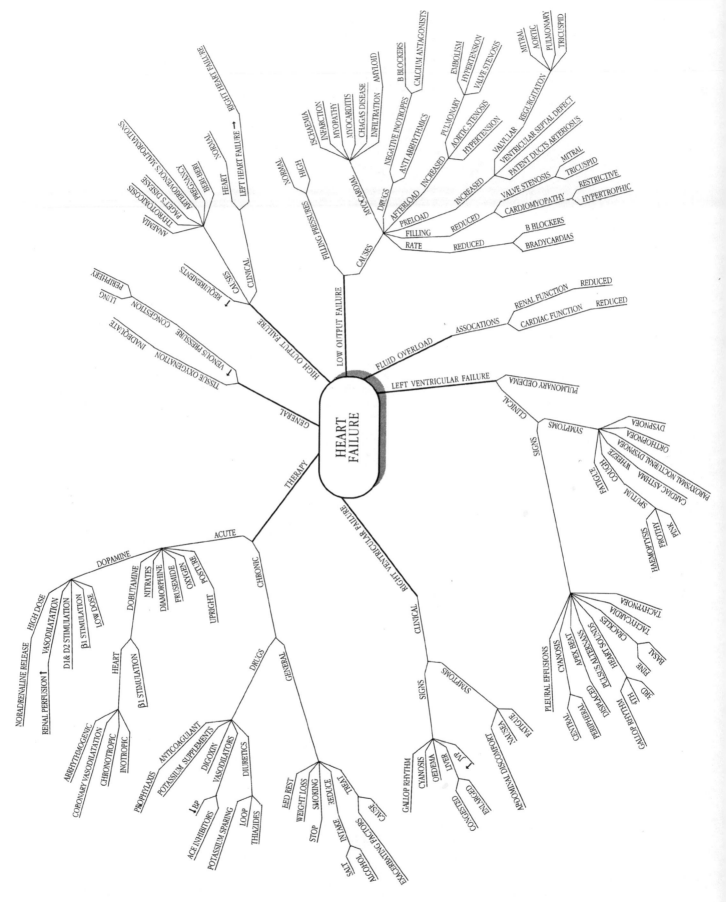

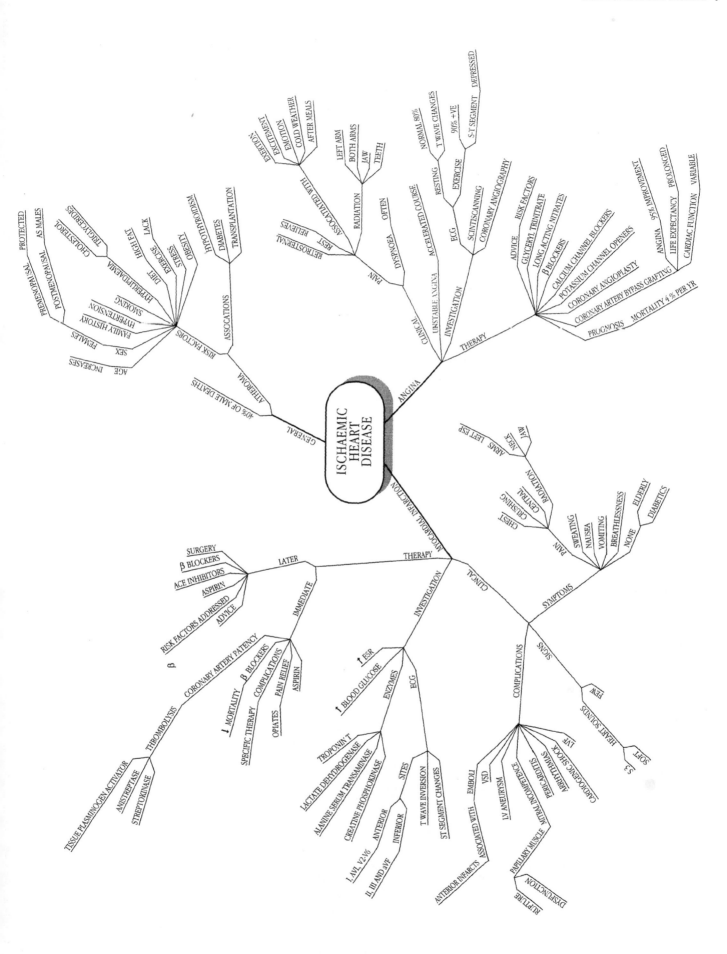

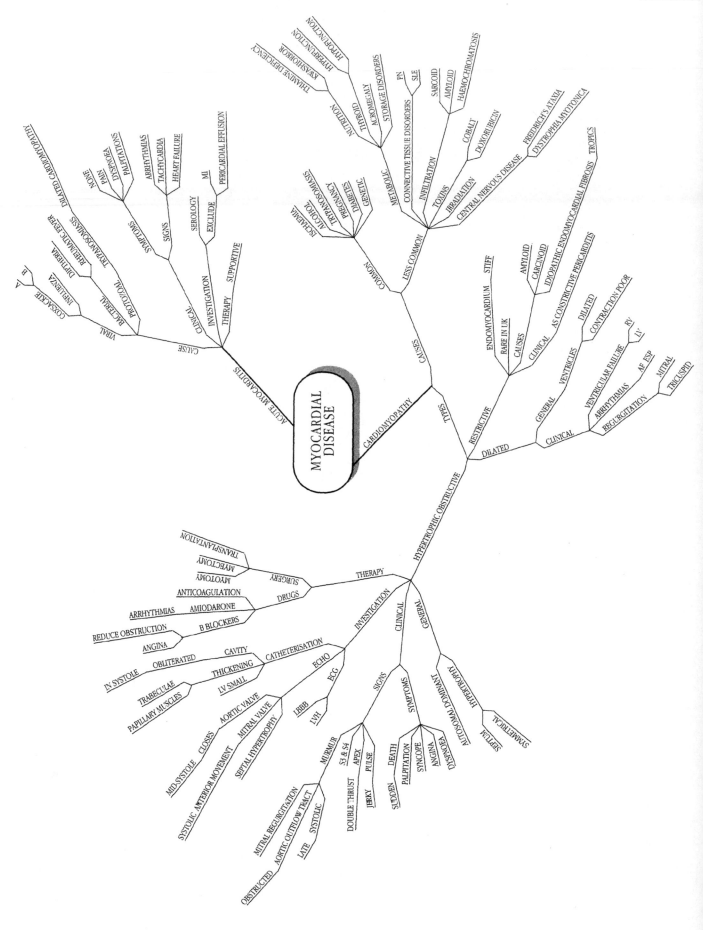

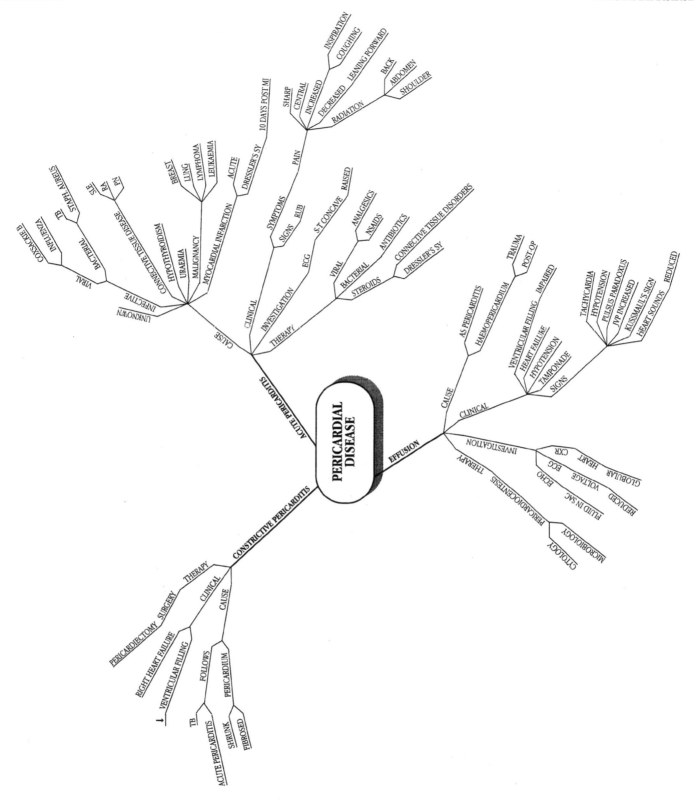

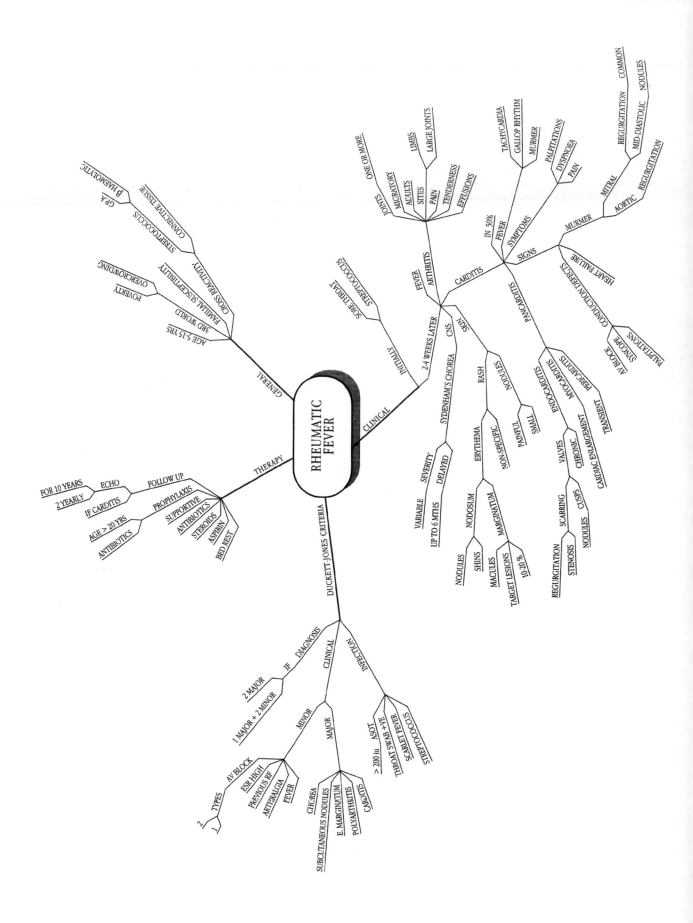

RHEUMATIC FEVER

GENERAL
- AGE 5-15 YRS
- 3RD WORLD
  - POVERTY
  - OVERCROWDING
- FAMILIAL SUSCEPTIBILITY
  - CROSS REACTIVITY
- STREPTOCOCCUS
  - CONNECTIVE TISSUE
  - GP A
  - β HAEMOLYTIC

CLINICAL
- INITIALLY
  - SORE THROAT
  - STREPTOCOCCUS
- 2-4 WEEKS LATER
  - FEVER
  - ARTHRITIS
    - JOINTS
      - ONE OR MORE
    - MIGRATORY
      - SITES
      - LIMBS
      - LARGE JOINTS
    - ADULTS
      - PAIN
      - TENDERNESS
      - EFFUSIONS
  - CARDITIS
    - IN 50%
    - FEVER
    - SYMPTOMS
      - TACHYCARDIA
      - GALLOP RHYTHM
      - MURMUR
      - PALPITATIONS
      - DYSPNOEA
      - PAIN
    - SIGNS
      - MURMER
        - MITRAL
          - REGURGITATION
          - COMMON
          - MID-DIASTOLIC
          - NODULES
        - AORTIC
          - REGURGITATION
      - HEART FAILURE
      - CONDUCTION DEFECTS
        - AV BLOCK
        - SYNCOPE
        - PALPITATIONS
    - PANCARDITIS
      - ENDOCARDITIS
        - VALVES
          - REGURGITATION
          - STENOSIS
          - NODULES
        - CHRONIC
          - SCARRING
          - CUSPS
      - MYOCARDITIS
        - CARDIAC ENLARGEMENT
      - PERICARDITIS
        - TRANSIENT
  - CNS
    - SYDENHAM'S CHOREA
      - SEVERITY
        - VARIABLE
      - DELAYED
        - UP TO 6 MTHS
  - SKIN
    - RASH
      - ERYTHEMA
        - NODOSUM
          - NODULES
          - SHINS
        - MARGINATUM
          - MACULES
          - TARGET LESIONS
          - 10-20 %
      - NON-SPECIFIC
    - NODULES
      - PAINFUL
      - SMALL

THERAPY
- FOLLOW UP
  - ECHO
    - FOR 10 YEARS
    - 2 YEARLY
    - IF CARDITIS
- PROPHYLAXIS
  - ANTIBIOTICS
    - AGE > 20 YRS
    - ANTIBIOTICS
- SUPPORTIVE
  - STEROIDS
  - ASPIRIN
  - BED REST

DUCKETT-JONES CRITERIA
- DIAGNOSIS
  - IF
    - 2 MAJOR
    - 1 MAJOR + 2 MINOR
- CLINICAL
  - MINOR
    - TYPES
      - 2
      - 1
    - AV BLOCK
    - ESR HIGH
    - PREVIOUS RF
    - ARTHRALGIA
    - FEVER
  - MAJOR
    - CHOREA
    - SUBCUTANEOUS NODULES
    - E. MARGINATUM
    - POLYARTHRITIS
    - CARDITIS
- INFECTION
  - ASOT
    - > 200 iu
  - THROAT SWAB +VE
  - SCARLET FEVER
  - STREPTOCOCCUS

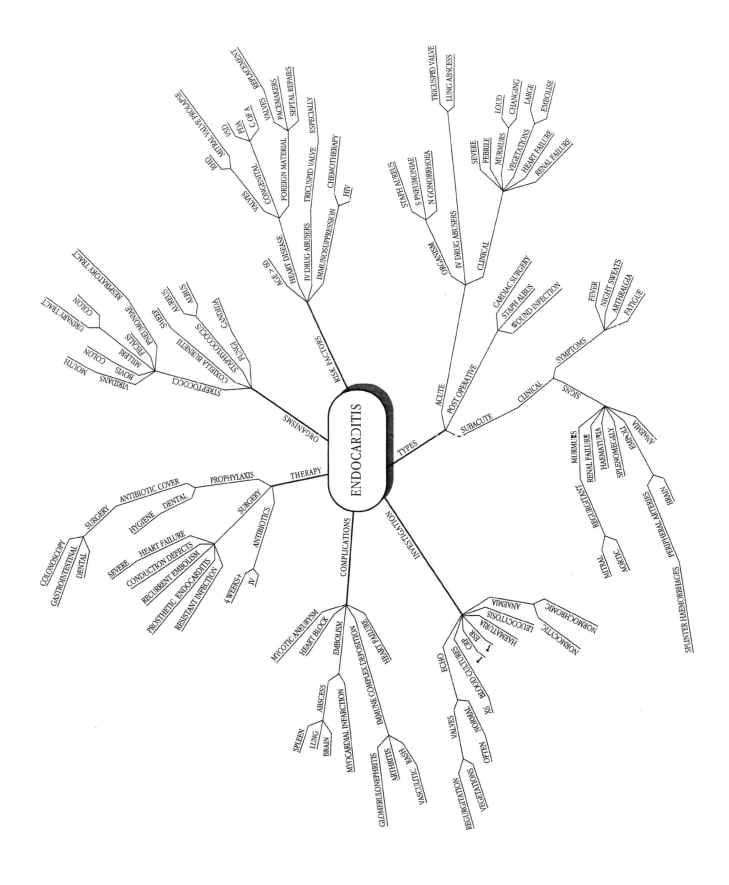

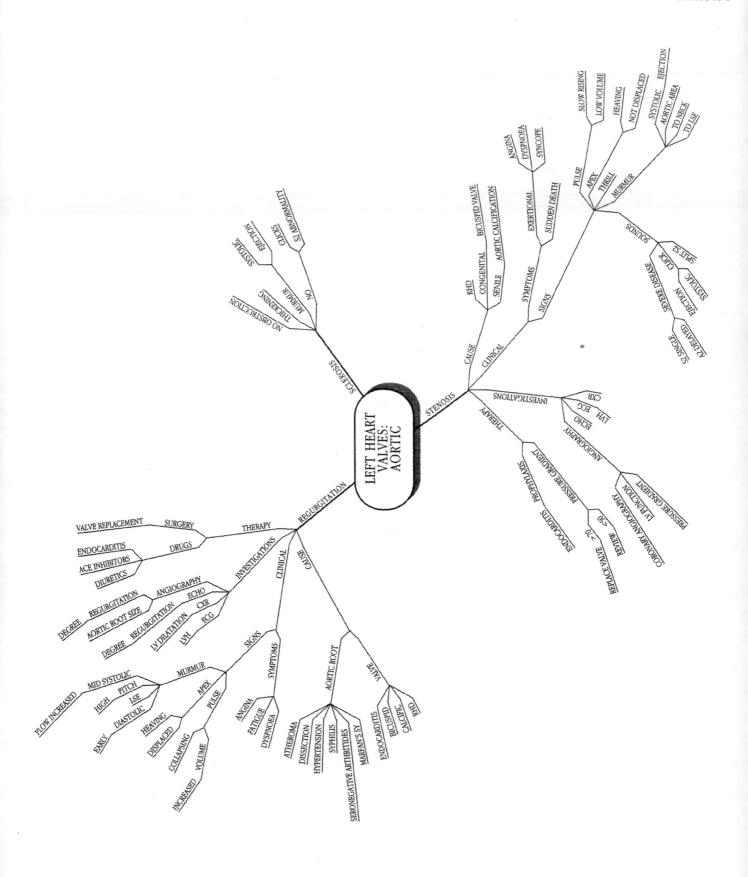

LEFT HEART VALVES: AORTIC

SCLEROSIS
- NO OBSTRUCTION
- MURMUR
  - NO
  - SYSTOLIC EJECTION
  - CLICKS
  - S2 ABNORMALITY
- THICKENING

STENOSIS
- CAUSE
  - RHD
  - CONGENITAL
  - BICUSPID VALVE
  - SENILE
  - AORTIC CALCIFICATION
- CLINICAL
  - SYMPTOMS
    - ANGINA
    - DYSPNOEA
    - SYNCOPE
    - EXERTIONAL
    - SUDDEN DEATH
  - SIGNS
    - PULSE
      - SLOW RISING
      - LOW VOLUME
    - APEX
      - HEAVING
      - NOT DISPLACED
    - THRILL
      - SYSTOLIC
      - AORTIC AREA
    - MURMUR
      - EJECTION
      - TO NECK
      - TO LSE
    - SOUNDS
      - SEVERE DISEASE
        - A2 DELAYED
        - SINGLE S2
      - EJECTION CLICK
      - SYSTOLIC
      - SPLIT S2
- INVESTIGATIONS
  - CXR
  - ECG
  - LVH
  - ECHO
  - ANGIOGRAPHY
    - PRESSURE GRADIENT
    - LV FUNCTION
    - CORONARY ANGIOGRAPHY
    - PRESSURE GRADIENT
      - REVIEW
      - < 50
      - > 70
      - REPLACE VALVE
- THERAPY
  - PROPHYLAXIS
    - ENDOCARDITIS

REGURGITATION
- CAUSE
  - VALVE
    - RHD
    - CALCIFIC
    - BICUSPID
    - ENDOCARDITIS
  - AORTIC ROOT
    - MARFAN'S SY
    - SYPHILIS
    - SERONEGATIVE ARTHRITIDES
    - HYPERTENSION
    - DISSECTION
    - ATHEROMA
- CLINICAL
  - SYMPTOMS
    - ANGINA
    - FATIGUE
    - DYSPNOEA
  - SIGNS
    - PULSE
      - COLLAPSING
      - VOLUME
      - INCREASED
    - APEX
      - HEAVING
      - DISPLACED
    - MURMUR
      - MID SYSTOLIC
        - FLOW INCREASED
      - PITCH
        - HIGH
      - LSE
      - DIASTOLIC
        - EARLY
- INVESTIGATIONS
  - ECHO
    - LV DILATATION
    - CXR
    - ECG
    - LVH
  - ANGIOGRAPHY
    - DEGREE
    - REGURGITATION
    - AORTIC ROOT SIZE
    - DEGREE
    - REGURGITATION
- THERAPY
  - DRUGS
    - ENDOCARDITIS
    - ACE INHIBITORS
    - DIURETICS
  - SURGERY
    - VALVE REPLACEMENT

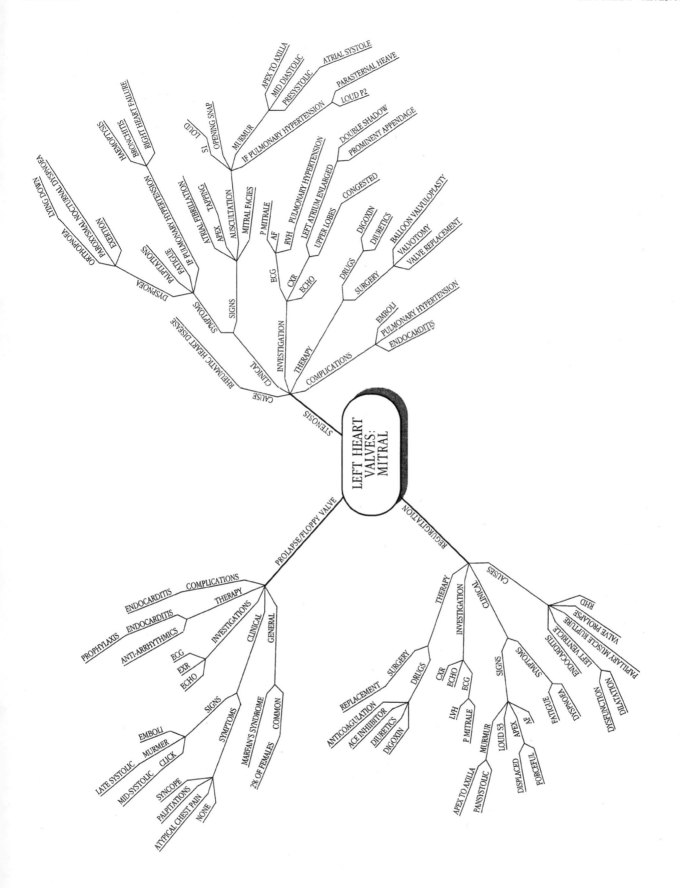

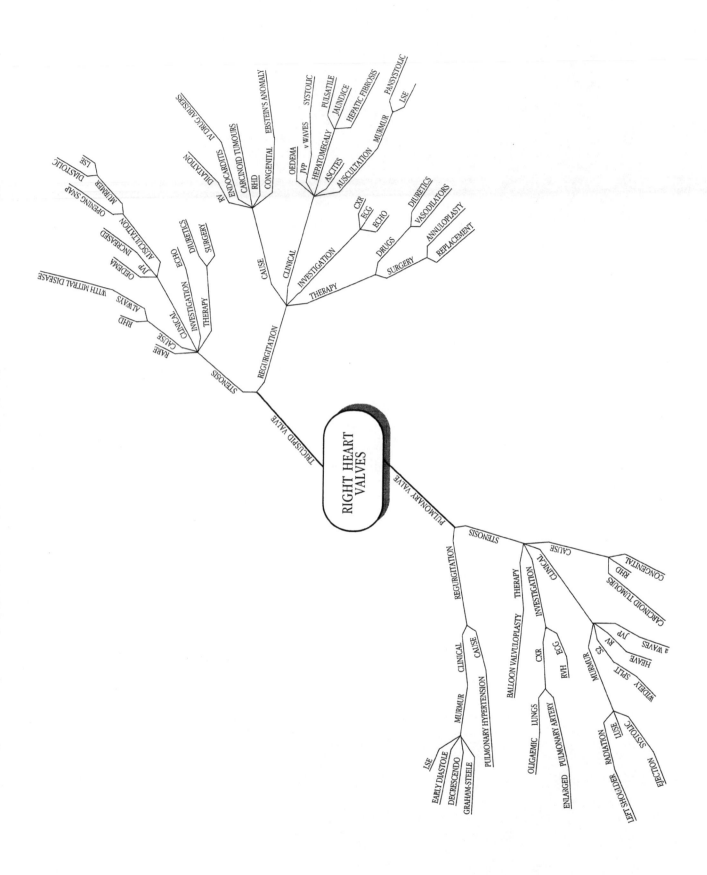

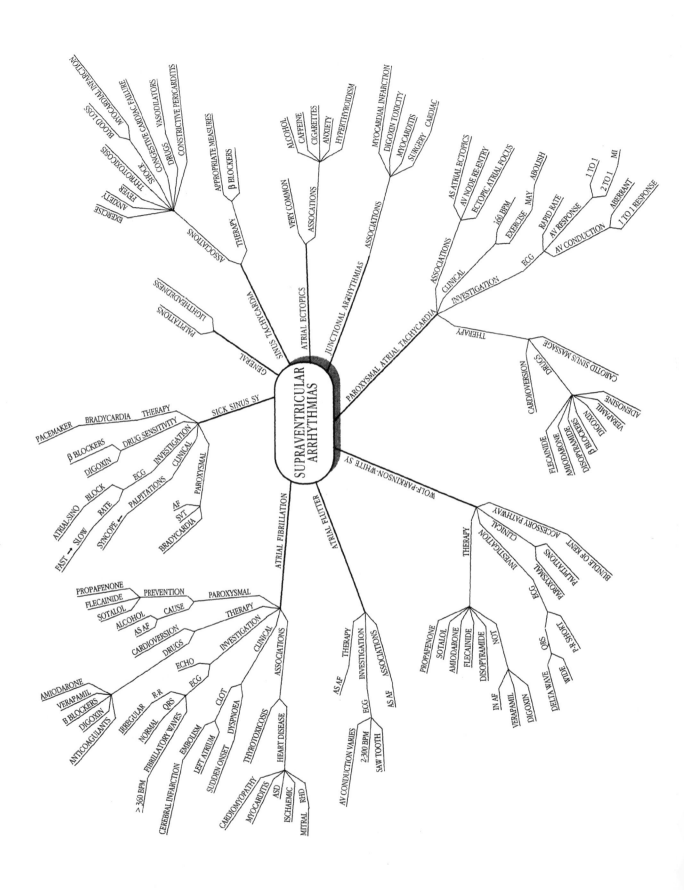

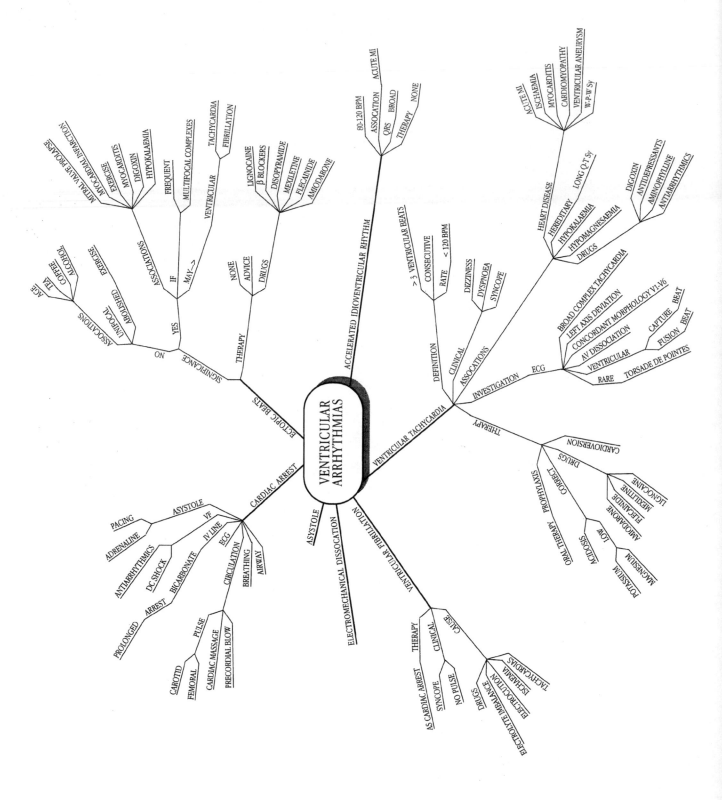

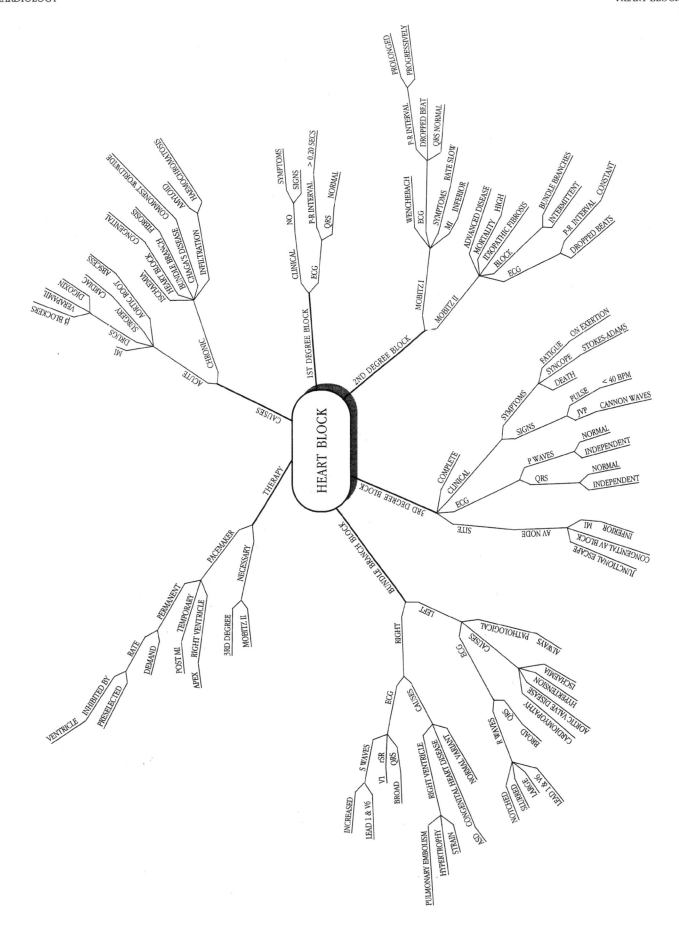

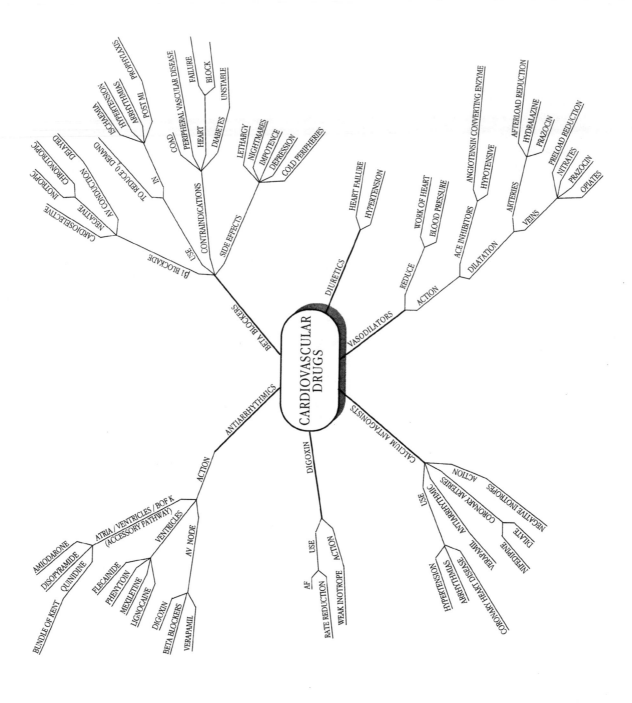

CARDIOVASCULAR DRUGS

BETA BLOCKERS
- β₁ BLOCKADE
  - CARDIOSELECTIVE
  - INOTROPIC — NEGATIVE
  - CHRONOTROPIC — NEGATIVE
    - AV CONDUCTION
    - DELAYED
  - TO REDUCE O₂ DEMAND
- USE
  - IN
    - ISCHAEMIA
    - HYPERTENSION
    - ARRHYTHMIAS
    - POST MI
    - PROPHYLAXIS
  - CONTRAINDICATIONS
    - COAD
    - PERIPHERAL VASCULAR DISEASE
    - HEART
      - FAILURE
      - BLOCK
    - DIABETES
    - UNSTABLE
  - SIDE EFFECTS
    - LETHARGY
    - NIGHTMARES
    - IMPOTENCE
    - DEPRESSION
    - COLD PERIPHERIES

DIURETICS
- HEART FAILURE
- HYPERTENSION

VASODILATORS
- REDUCE
  - WORK OF HEART
  - BLOOD PRESSURE
- ACTION
  - ACE INHIBITORS
    - ANGIOTENSIN CONVERTING ENZYME
    - HYPOTENSIVE
  - DILATATION
    - ARTERIES
      - AFTERLOAD REDUCTION
        - HYDRALAZINE
        - PRAZOCIN
    - VEINS
      - PRELOAD REDUCTION
        - NITRATES
        - PRAZOCIN
        - OPIATES

CALCIUM ANTAGONISTS
- ACTION
  - NEGATIVE INOTROPES
  - CORONARY ARTERIES
  - DILATE
    - NIFEDIPINE
    - VERAPAMIL
- USE
  - ANTIARRHYTHMIC
  - CORONARY HEART DISEASE
  - ARRHYTHMIAS
  - HYPERTENSION

DIGOXIN
- USE
  - AF
  - RATE REDUCTION
- ACTION
  - WEAK INOTROPE

ANTIARRHYTHMICS
- ACTION
  - ATRIA / VENTRICLES / BOF K (ACCESSORY PATHWAY)
    - AMIODARONE
    - DISOPYRAMIDE
    - QUINIDINE
    - BUNDLE OF KENT
  - VENTRICLES
    - FLECAINIDE
    - PHENYTOIN
    - MEXILETINE
    - LIGNOCAINE
  - AV NODE
    - DIGOXIN
    - BETA BLOCKERS
    - VERAPAMIL

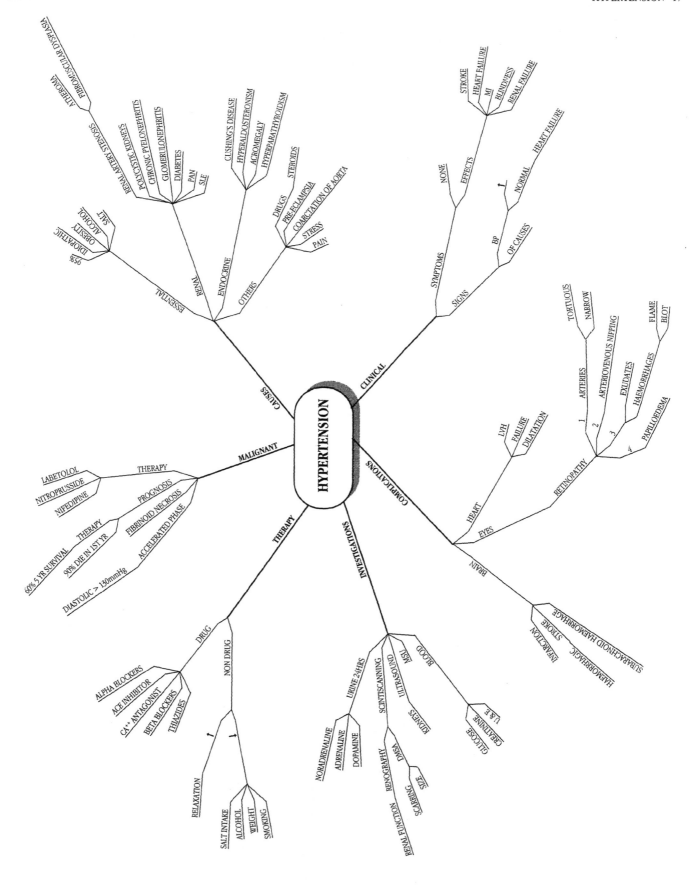

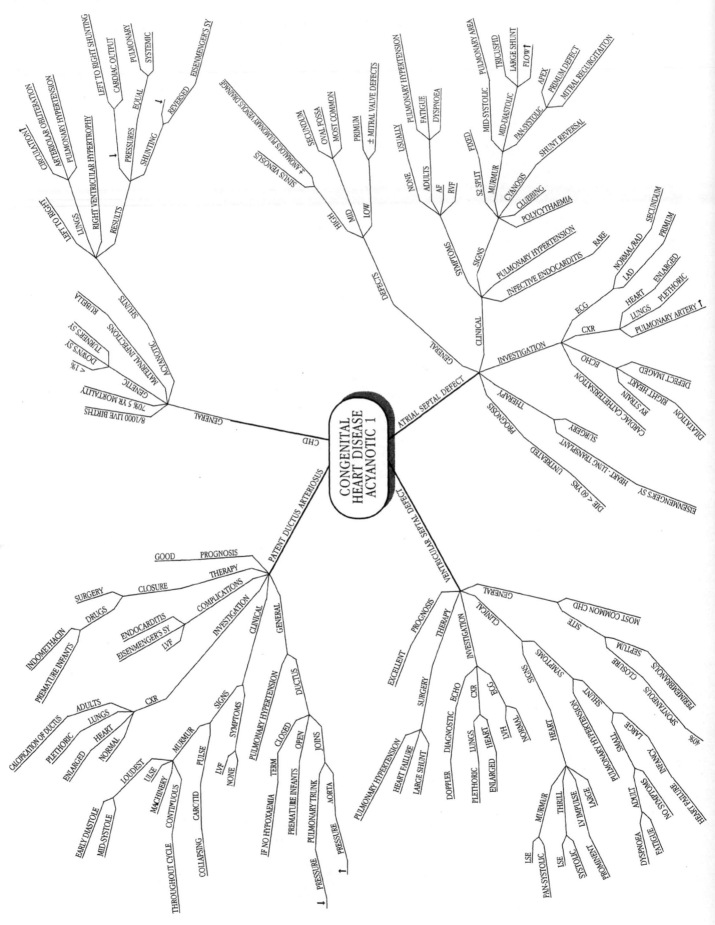

CONGENITAL HEART DISEASE ACYANOTIC 1

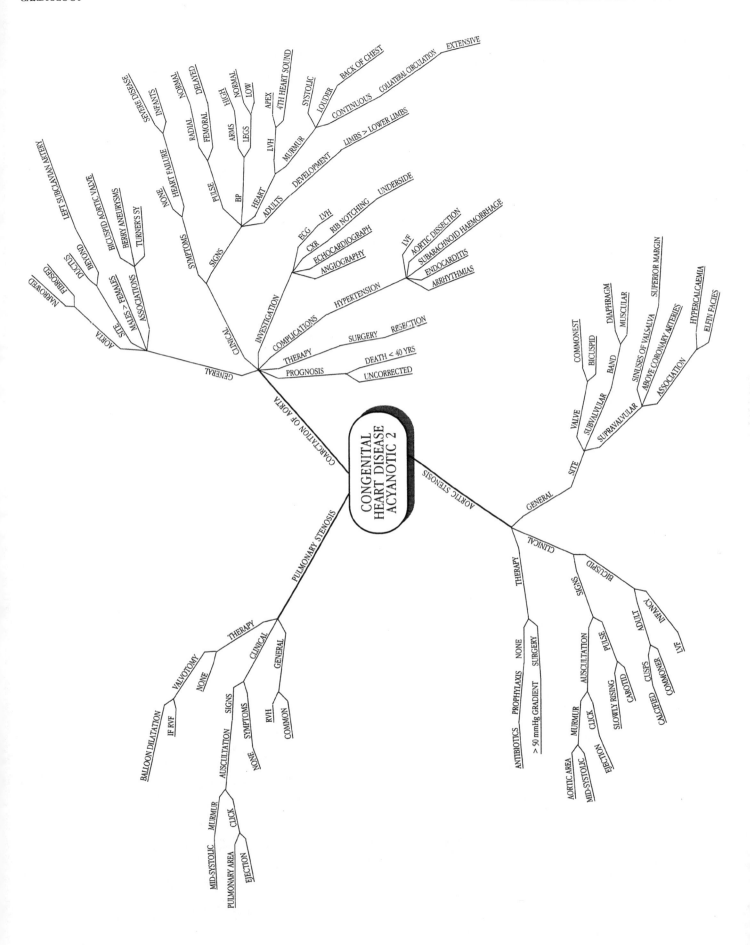

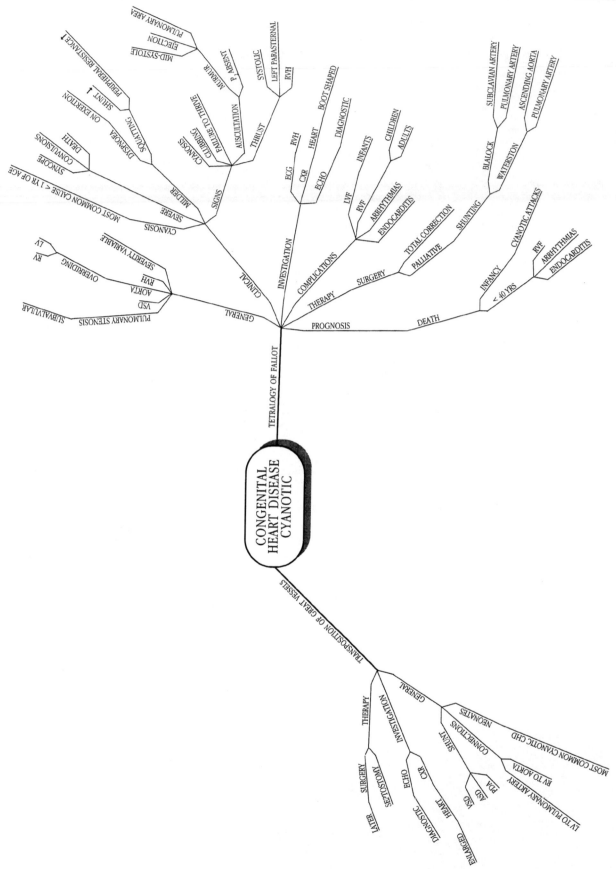

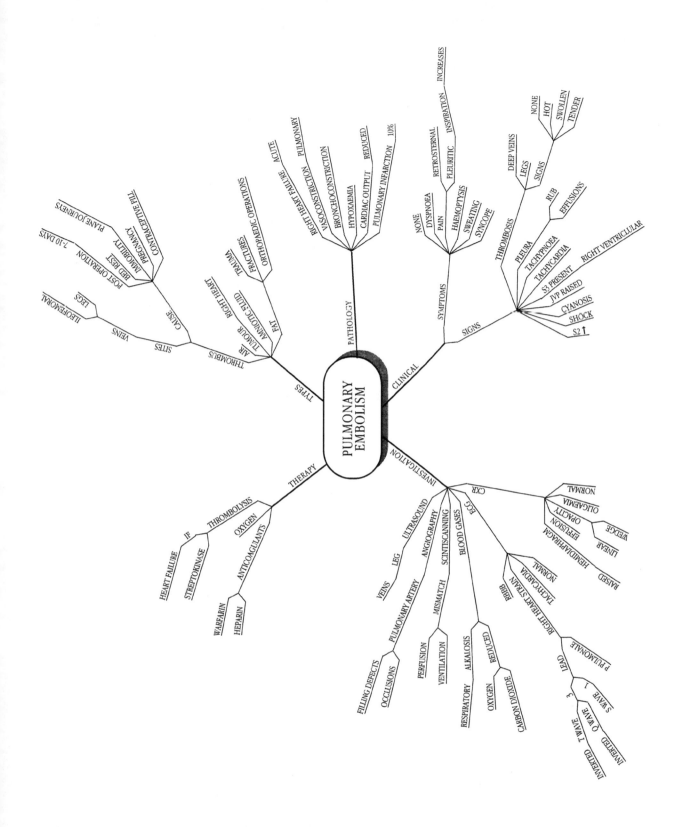

Respiratory system

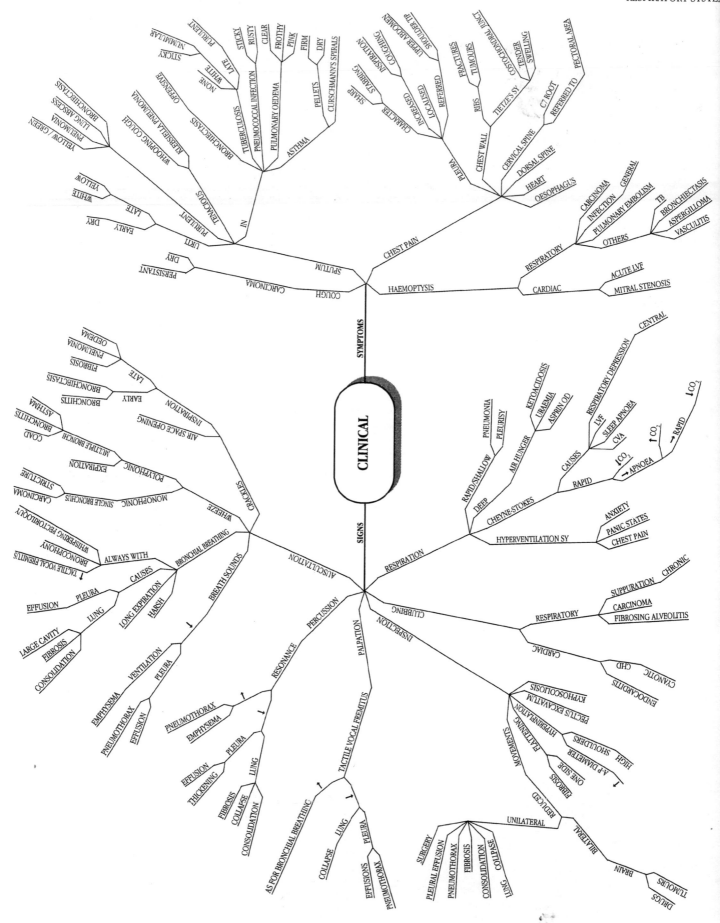

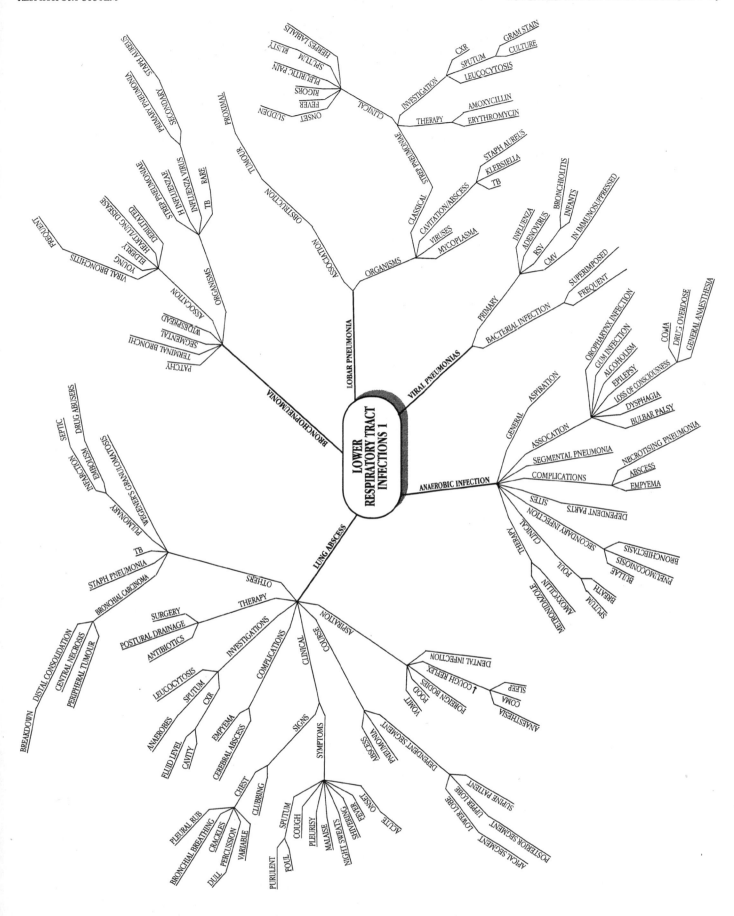

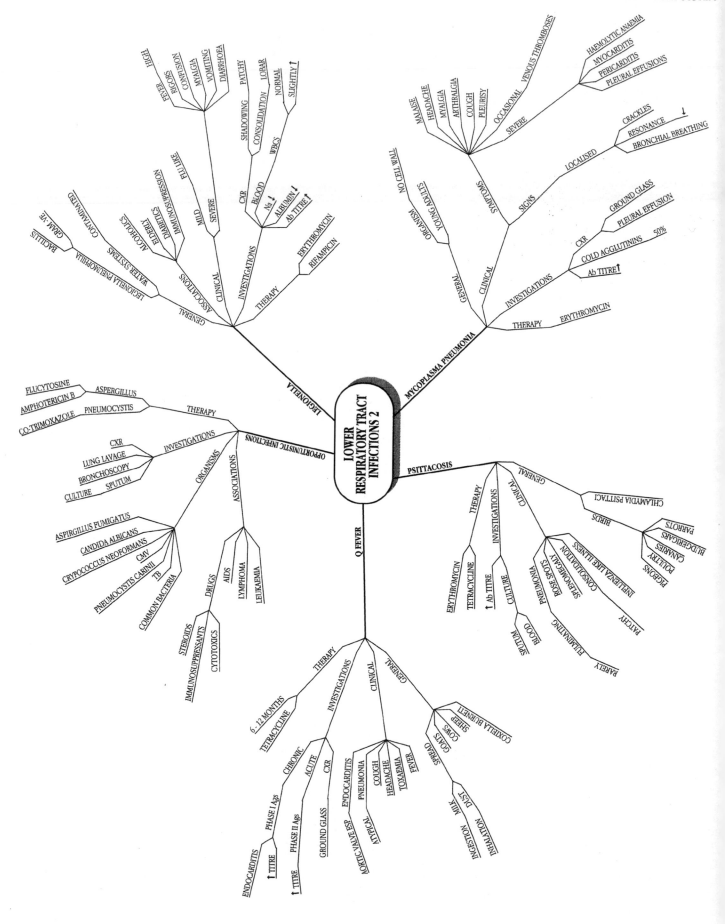

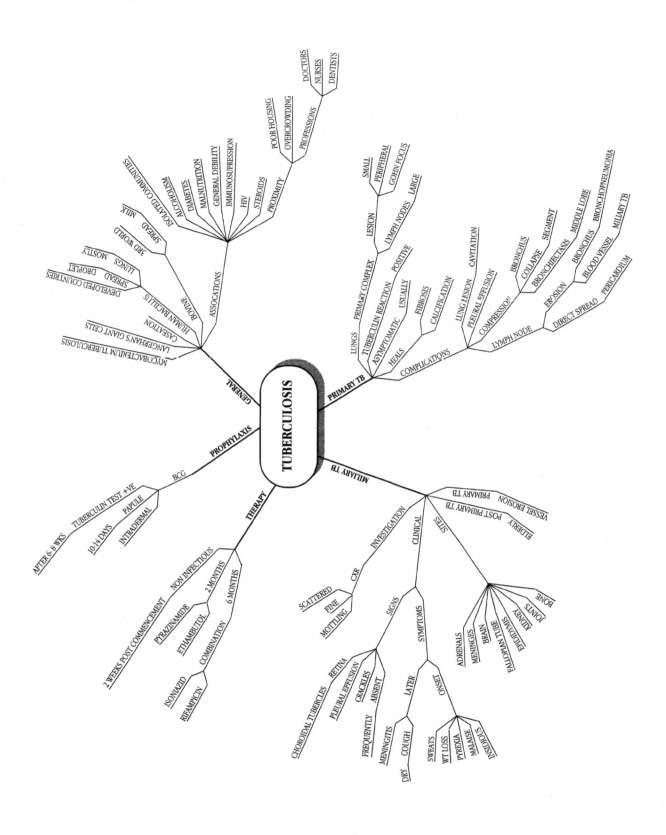

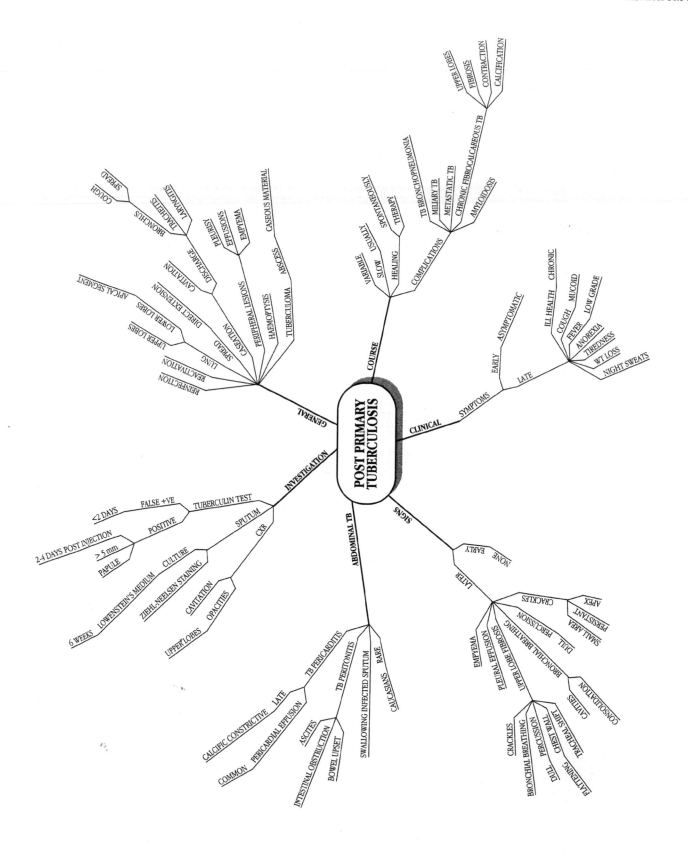

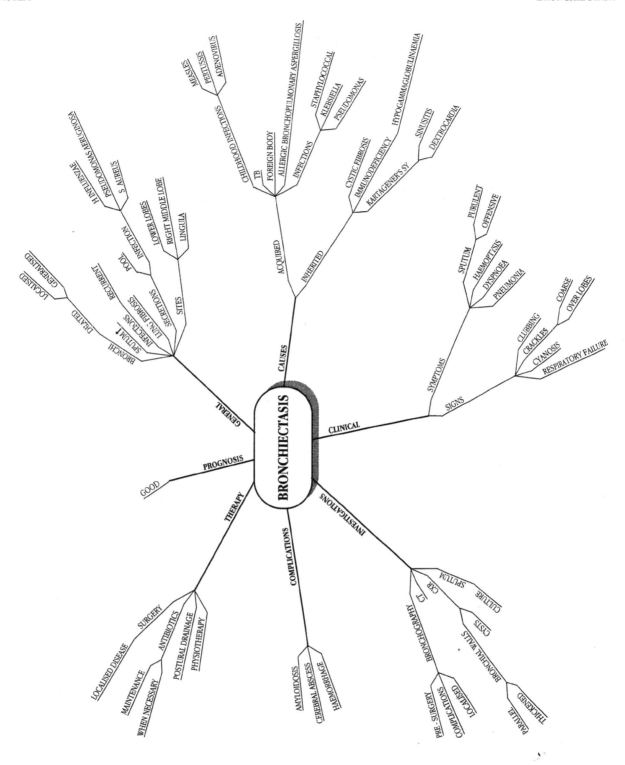

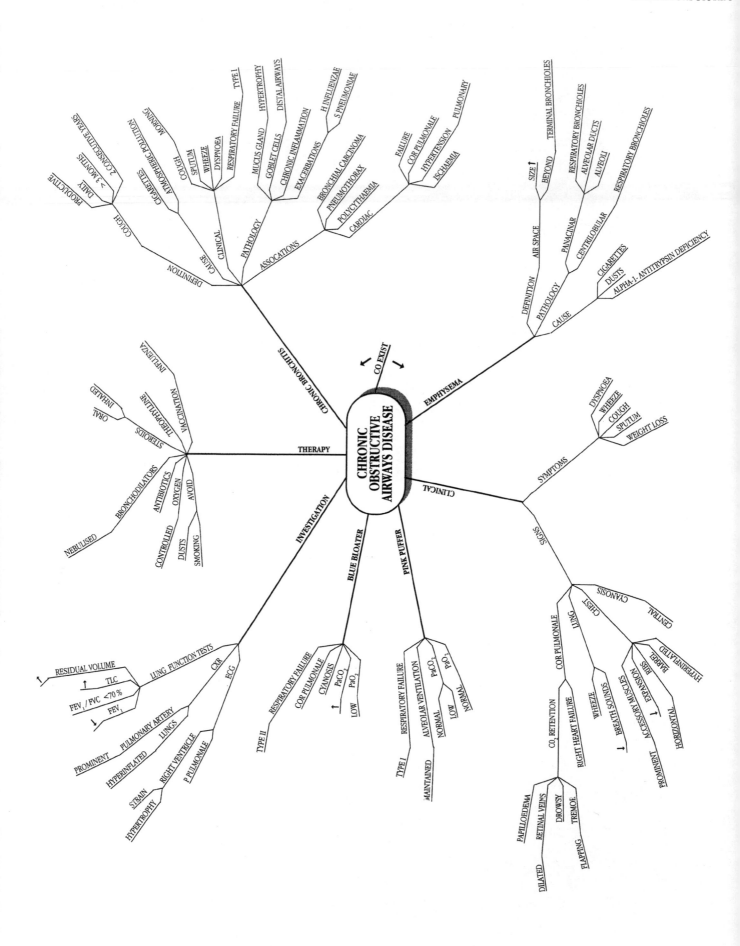

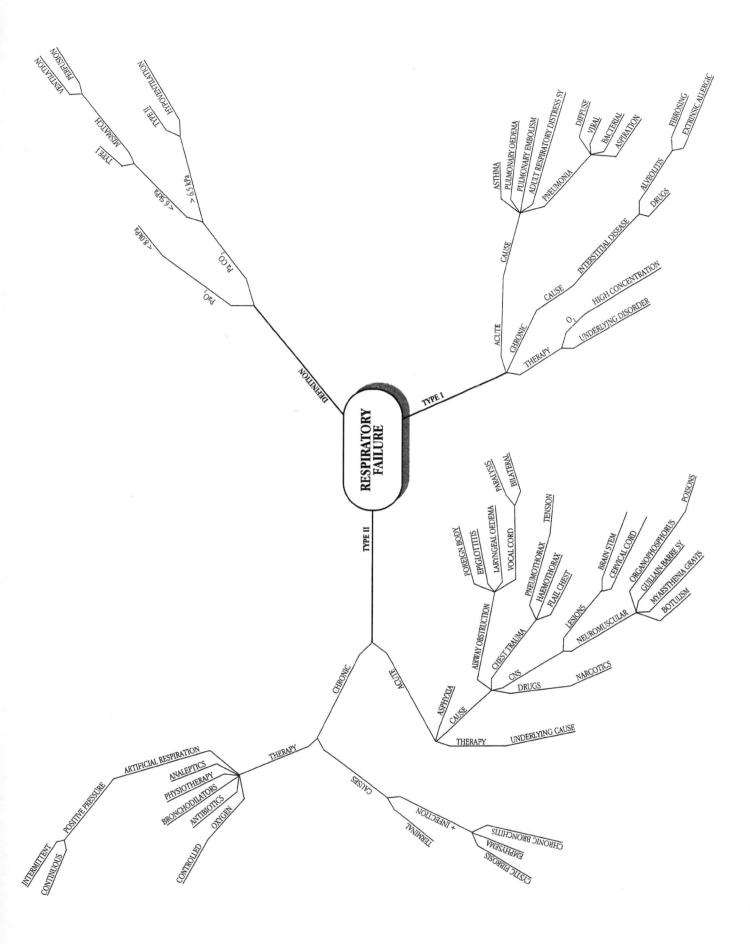

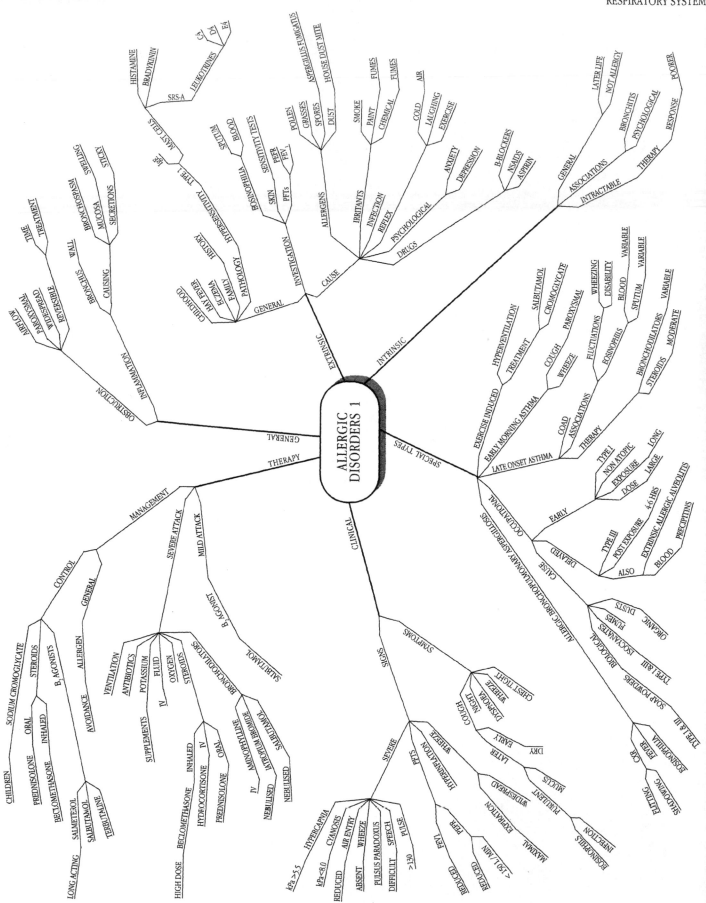

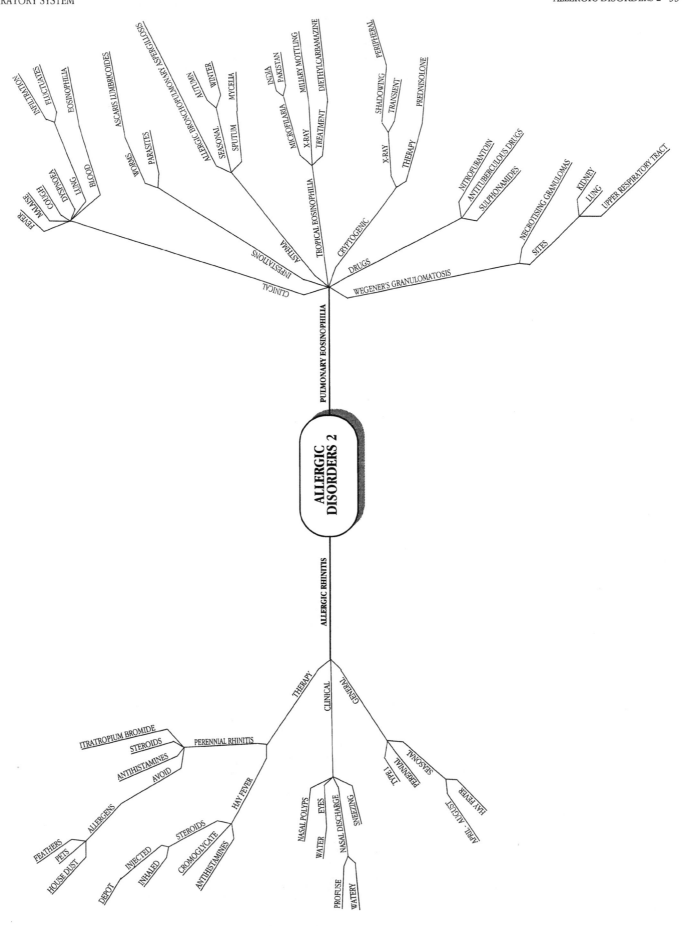

ALLERGIC DISORDERS 2

PULMONARY EOSINOPHILIA

CLINICAL
INFESTATIONS
FEVER
MALAISE
COUGH
DYSPNOEA
LUNG
BLOOD
INFILTRATION
FLUCTUATES
EOSINOPHILIA
WORMS
PARASITES
ASCARIS LUMBRICOIDES
ALLERGIC BRONCHOPULMONARY ASPERGILLOSIS
SEASONAL
AUTUMN
WINTER
MYCELIA
SPUTUM

ASTHMA

TROPICAL EOSINOPHILIA
MICROFILARIA
X-RAY
INDIA
PAKISTAN
MILIARY MOTTLING
TREATMENT
DIETHYLCARBAMAZINE

CRYPTOGENIC
X-RAY
SHADOWING
TRANSIENT
PERIPHERAL
THERAPY
PREDNISOLONE

DRUGS
NITROFURANTOIN
ANTITUBERCULOUS DRUGS
SULPHONAMIDES

WEGENER'S GRANULOMATOSIS
SITES
NECROTISING GRANULOMAS
KIDNEY
LUNG
UPPER RESPIRATORY TRACT

ALLERGIC RHINITIS

THERAPY
PERENNIAL RHINITIS
ITRATROPIUM BROMIDE
STEROIDS
ANTIHISTAMINES
AVOID
ALLERGENS
FEATHERS
PETS
HOUSE DUST

HAY FEVER
STEROIDS
DEPOT
INJECTED
INHALED
CROMOGLYCATE
ANTIHISTAMINES

CLINICAL
NASAL POLYPS
EYES
WATER
NASAL DISCHARGE
PROFUSE
WATERY
SNEEZING

GENERAL
TYPE I
PERENNIAL
SEASONAL
APRIL - AUGUST
HAY FEVER

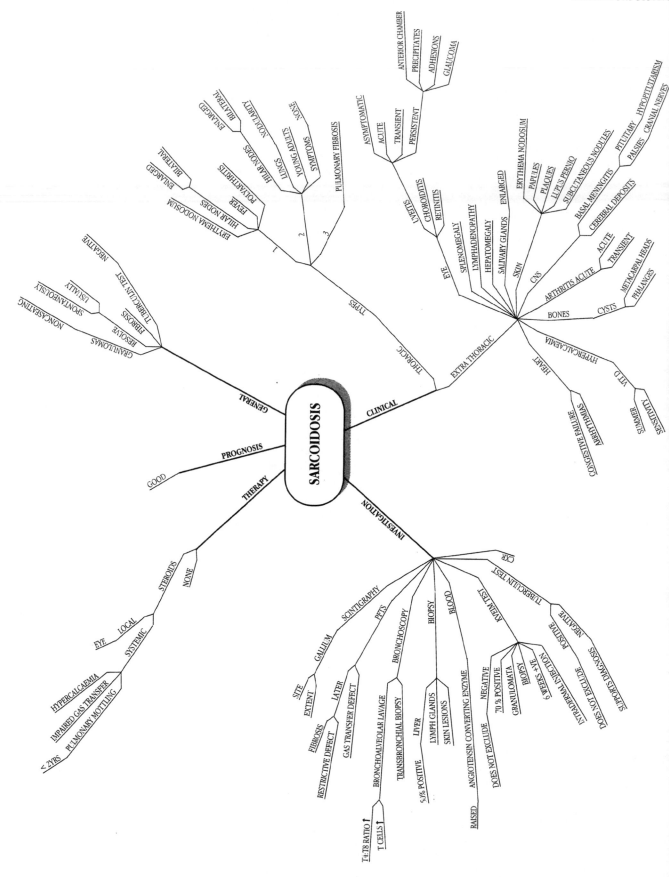

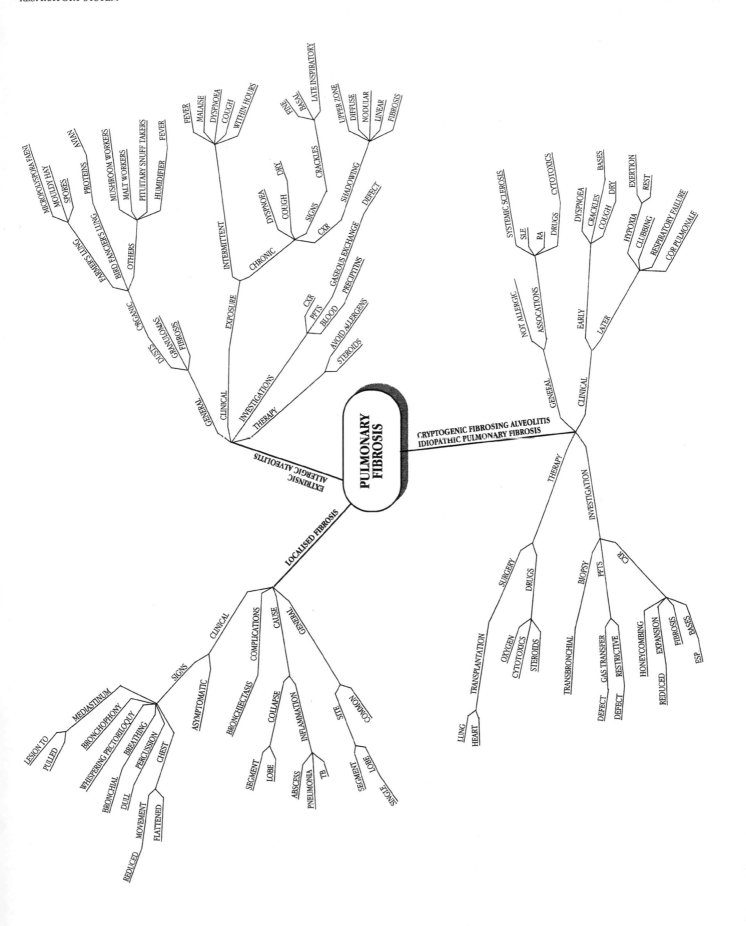

PULMONARY FIBROSIS

CRYPTOGENIC FIBROSING ALVEOLITIS
IDIOPATHIC PULMONARY FIBROSIS

EXTRINSIC ALLERGIC ALVEOLITIS

LOCALISED FIBROSIS

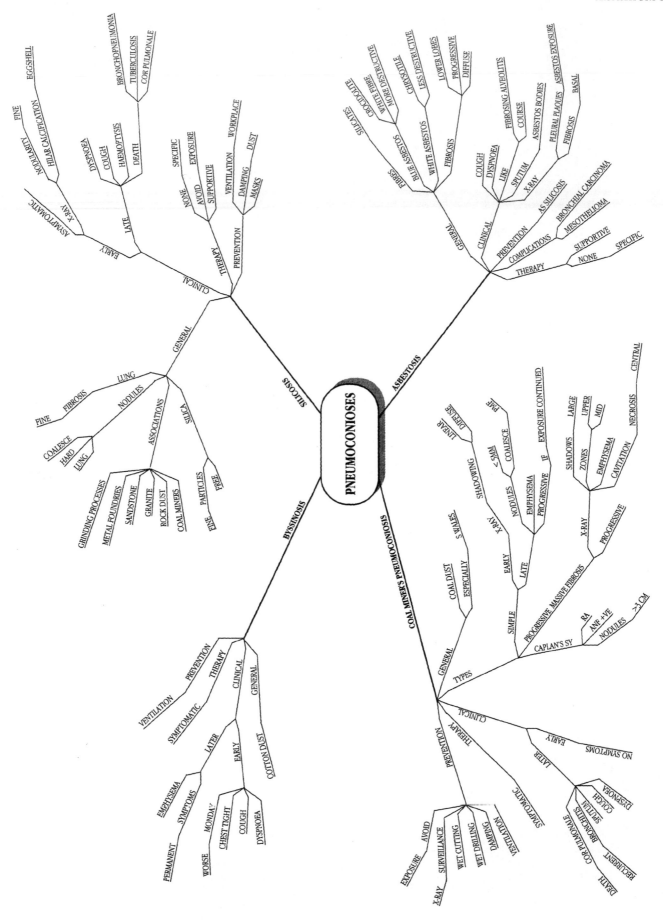

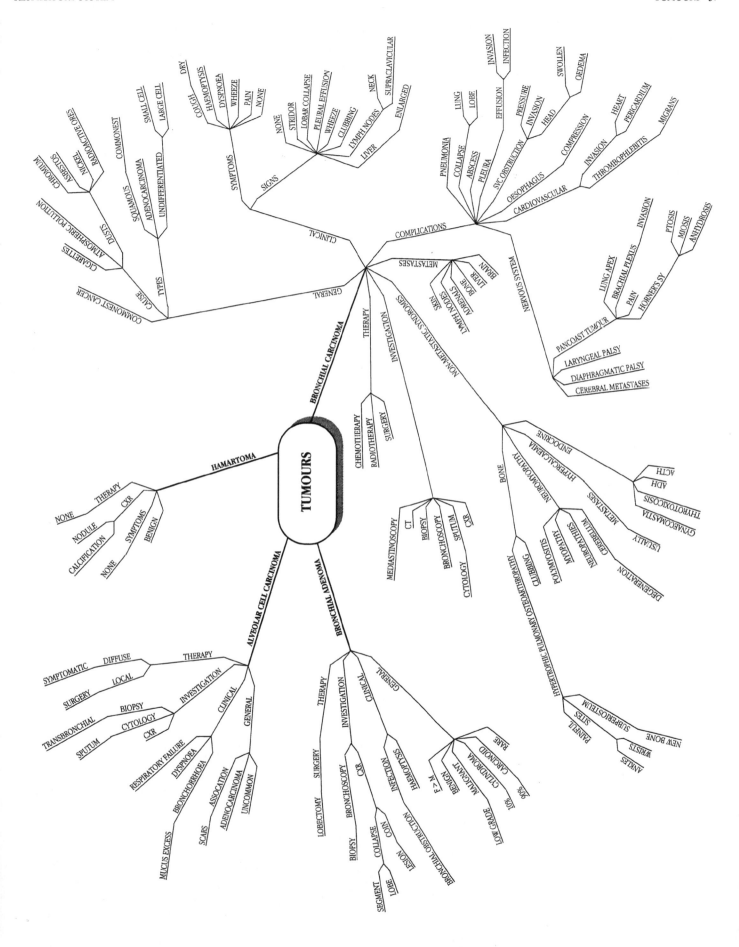

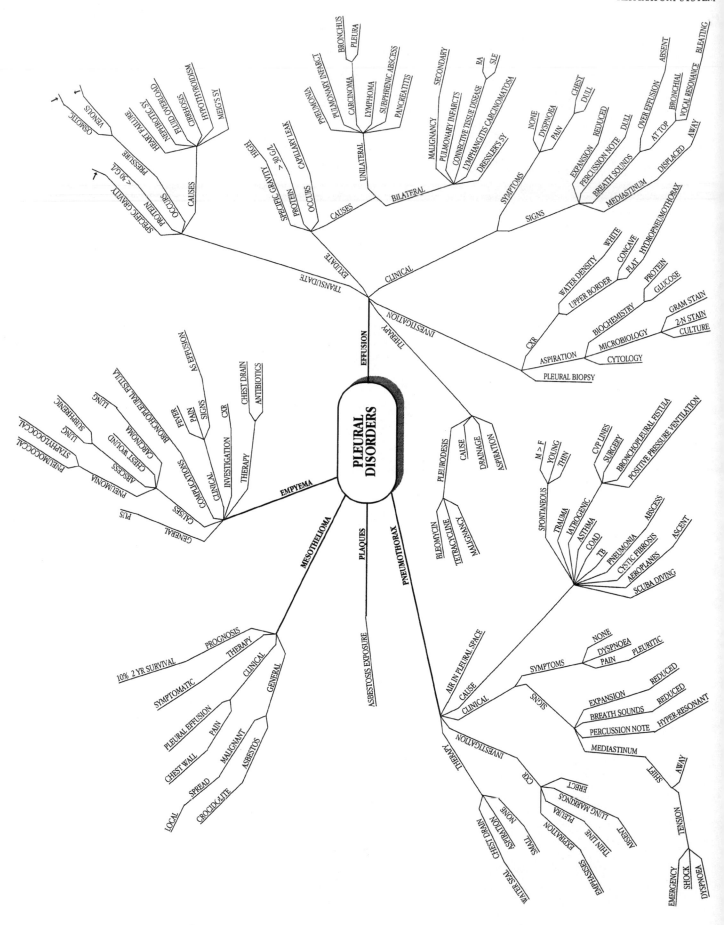

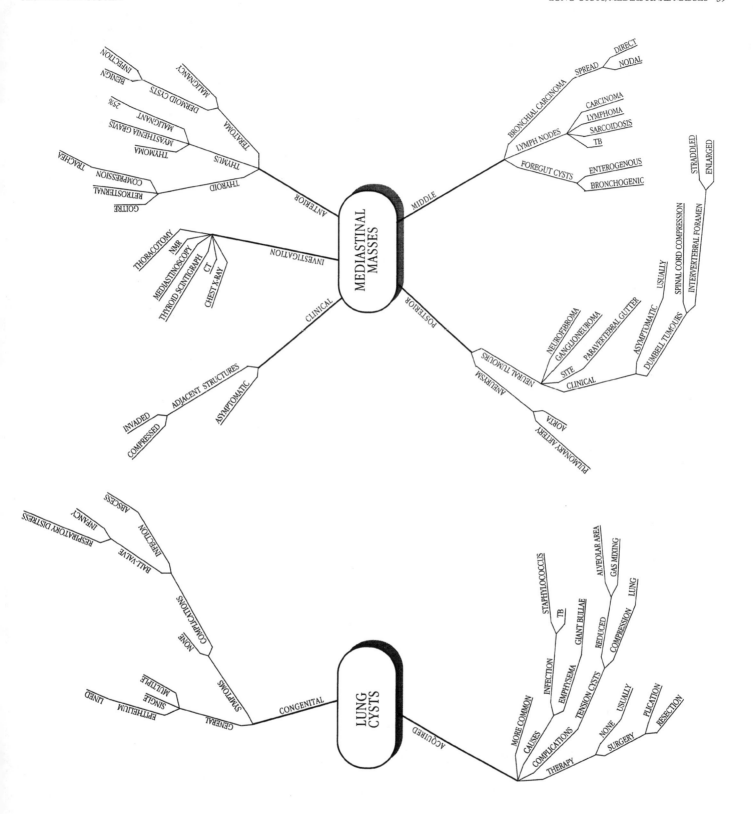

Central nervous system

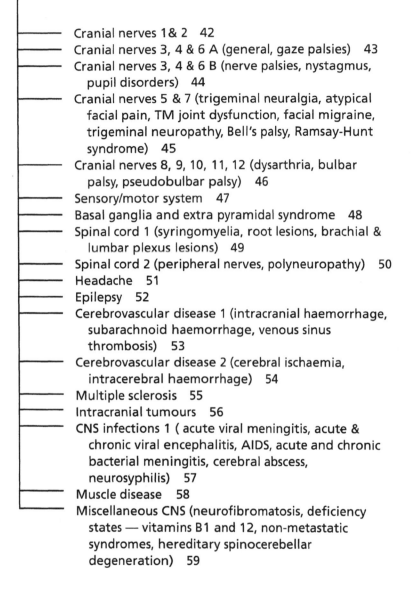

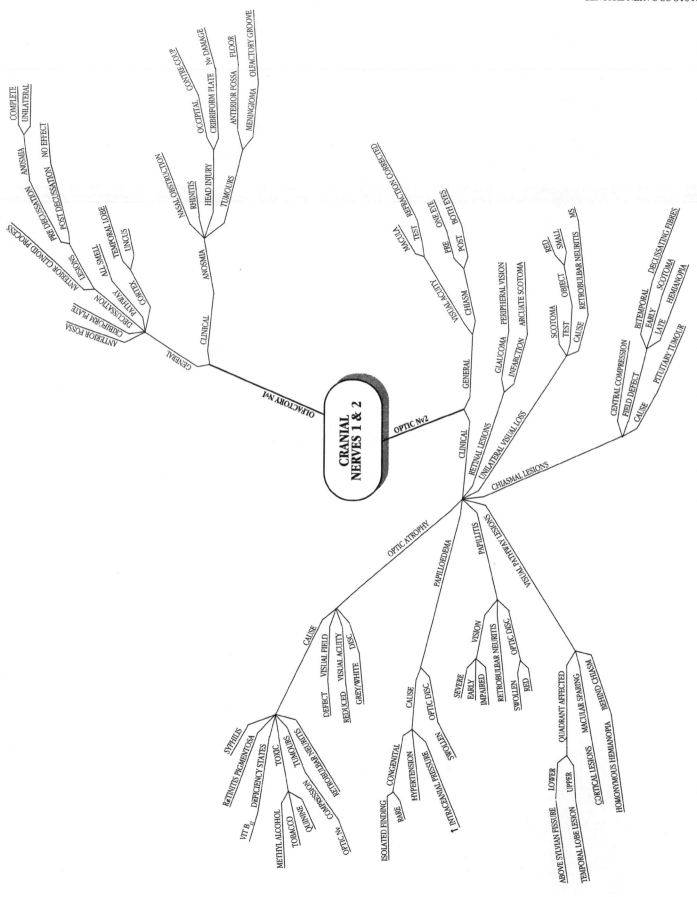

CRANIAL NERVES 3, 4 & 6 A

GENERAL

- SUPPLY
  - EXTERNAL OCULAR MUSCLES
  - LEVATOR PALPEBRAE
  - PARASYMPATHETIC
  - SMOOTH MUSCLE
- ANATOMY
  - 3
    - EMERGES — MIDBRAIN — VENTRAL — INTERPEDUNCULAR FOSSA
    - LEAVES — POST CEREBELLAR ARTERY (ABOVE) / SUPERIOR CEREBELLAR (BELOW) — LATERAL
    - POSTERIOR CLINOID PROCESS
    - CAVERNOUS SINUS
    - SUPERIOR ORBITAL FISSURE
    - BRANCHES — SUPERIOR / INFERIOR
      - SUP RECTUS M / LEVATOR PALPEBRAE
      - RECTI (MEDIAL / INFERIOR) / INF OBLIQUE M / CILIARY GANGLION — PARASYMPATHETIC
    - LOWER BORDER
  - 4
    - EMERGES — PONS — VENTRAL
    - CAVERNOUS SINUS
    - SUPERIOR ORBITAL FISSURE — SYMPATHETIC FIBRES JOIN — LATERAL RECTUS M
    - SUPERIOR OBLIQUE M
  - 6
    - EMERGES — BRAINSTEM — DORSAL
    - RUNS VENTRALLY
    - CAVERNOUS SINUS — SYMPATHETIC FIBRES JOIN
    - S ORBITAL FISSURE
- LESIONS
  - INTRAMEDULLARY — ASSOCIATION — LONG TRACT SIGNS — LIMBS
  - EXTRAMEDULLARY
    - 5, 6, 7 & 8
    - INCOORDINATION — IPSILATERAL — CEREBELLAR
    - LESION — CEREBELLOPONTINE ANGLE

GAZE PALSIES

- SUPRANUCLEAR
  - INTERNUCLEAR OPTHALMOPLEGIA
    - LESION — MEDIAL LONGDITUDINAL FASCICULUS — COMMON — MS
    - PARALYSIS — IPSILATERAL
    - CONVERGENCE — NORMAL
    - AFFECTS — 6 (SPARES) / 3
    - CONTRALATERAL / IPSILATERAL
  - PONS
    - PARALYSIS — RARE
    - HORIZONTAL CONJUGATE MOVEMENT
  - MIDBRAIN
    - PARALYSIS — RARE
    - VERTICAL CONJUGATE MOVEMENT
    - CONVERGENCE
  - BRAINSTEM
    - FUNCTION — INTACT
    - REFLEX CONJUGATE MOVEMENT
      - DOLL'S HEAD MOVEMENT
      - CALORIC TEST — NORMAL
  - CLINICAL
    - PARALYSIS — CONJUGATE
    - EYES DEVIATE TO SIDE OF LESION
    - TO CONTRALATERAL SIDE
  - CAUSES
    - COMMON — CEREBRAL HEMISPHERE — PREMOTOR-FRONTAL CORTEX
    - STROKE — LARGE
    - HEAD INJURY — SEVERE

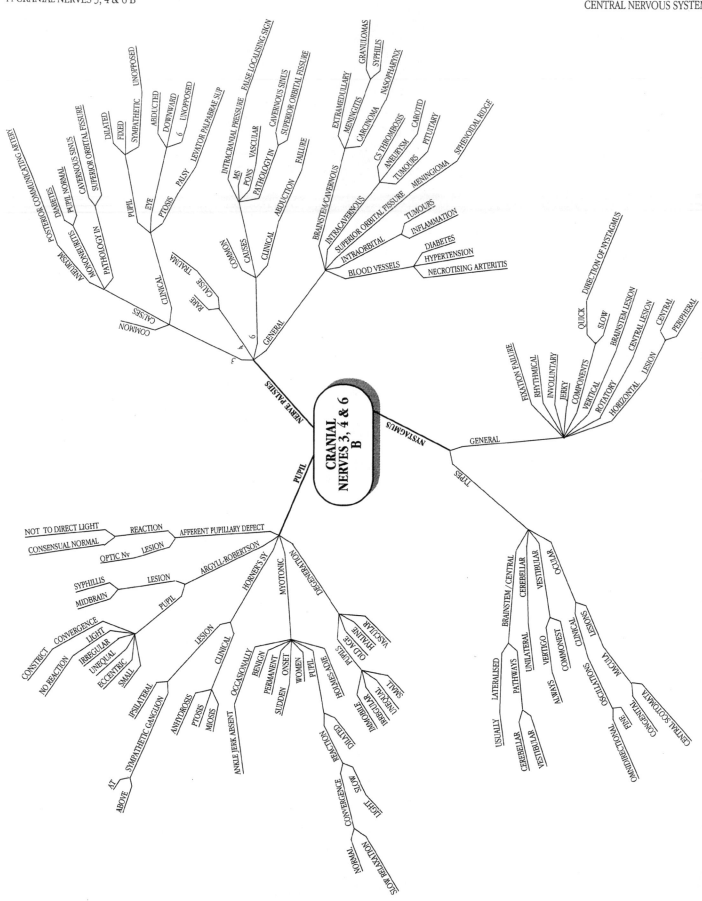

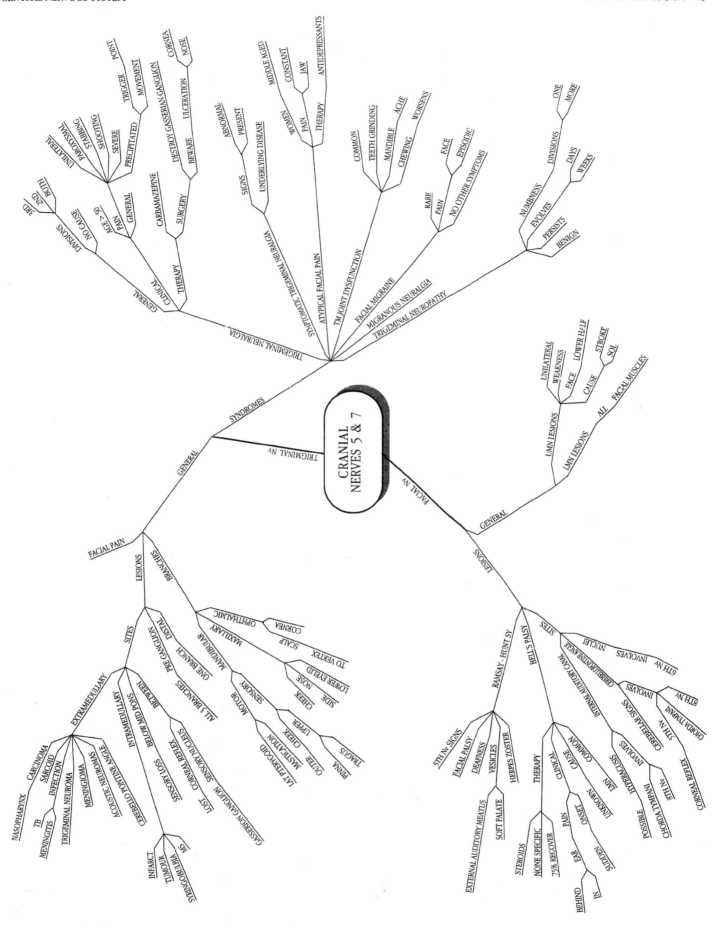

CRANIAL NERVES 8, 9, 10, 11 & 12

AUDITORY Nv 8

- ACOUSTIC Nv
  - GENERAL
    - ACOUSTIC
    - VESTIBULAR
    - COCHLEA
    - RELATIONS
      - OTOLITH
      - SEMICIRCULAR CANALS
      - AUDITORY CANAL
      - INFERIOR CEREBELLAR PEDUNCLE
      - CEREBELLOPONTINE ANGLE
      - AIR LOUDER
      - CHORDA TYMPANI
      - 7TH Nv
    - DEAFNESS
      - PERCEPTIVE
        - C-P ANGLE
          - TUMOURS
            - MAY INVOLVE
              - 5TH Nv
              - 7TH Nv
              - CEREBELLUM
            - PAGET'S DISEASE
              - MAY INVOLVE
                - TASTE IMPAIRED
        - TEMPORAL BONE
      - LESIONS
        - OTHER SIGNS
        - BRAINSTEM
      - CONNECTIONS
    - TEST
  - CLINICAL
    - VESTIBULAR NEURONITIS
      - CEREBELLUM
      - 3RD, 4TH & 6TH Nvs
      - VERTIGO
      - DYSEQUILIBRIUM
      - CALORIC
      - NYSTAGMUS
      - ACUTE
      - NAUSEA
      - NYSTAGMUS
      - GAIT
      - UNSTEADY
      - DURATION
        - DAYS
        - VERTIGO
        - WEEKS
    - MENIERE'S DISEASE
      - CAUSE
        - ↑ ENDOLYMPHATIC PRESSURE
      - CLINICAL
        - VERTIGO
        - TINNITUS
        - DEAFNESS
        - NYSTAGMUS
        - RECURRENT
        - PERSISTENT
        - PROGRESSIVE
        - DURING ATTACK
      - THERAPY
        - VASODILATORS
        - BETAHISTINE
        - PHENOTHIAZINES

GLOSSOPHARYNGEAL Nv 9

- VAGUS Nv
- ACCESSORY Nvs
- SENSORY
  - ALL SENSATION
    - TO
      - TONGUE
      - POSTERIOR
      - TONSILS
      - PHARYNX
- MOTOR
  - STYLOPHARYNGEUS M
- LESIONS
  - RARE
  - ISOLATED
  - JUGULAR FORAMEN
  - INVOLVES
- GLOSSOPHARYNGEAL NEURALGIA
  - SIMILAR TO TRIGEMINAL NEURALGIA

VAGUS Nv 10

- SENSORY
  - LARYNX
  - PHARYNX
- MOTOR
  - PHARYNX
  - LARYNX
- PARASYMPATHETIC
  - VISCERA
    - THORAX
    - ABDOMEN
    - SOFT PALATE
    - PHARYNX
    - LARYNX
- CLINICAL
  - PARALYSIS
    - PHONATION
    - UVULA
    - DEVIATION
    - CONTRALATERAL

ACCESSORY Nv 11

- MOTOR
  - STERNOMASTOID M
  - TRAPEZIUS M

HYPOGLOSSAL Nv 12

- MUSCLES
  - TONGUE
- CLINICAL
  - TONGUE
    - DEVIATION
    - WEAK
    - FASCICULATION
    - WASTING
    - IPSILATERAL
    - AFFECTED SIDE
  - CAUSES
    - MYASTHENIA GRAVIS
    - CEREBELLAR LESIONS
    - EXTRAPYRAMIDAL LESIONS
    - LMN
    - UMN
    - BULBAR PALSY
    - PSEUDOBULBAR PALSY

DYSARTHRIA

BULBAR PALSY

- CLINICAL
  - CAUSE
    - GENERAL
      - LMN
      - MEDULLARY
      - EXTRAMEDULLARY
      - LESION
        - MEDULLA
        - BULB
    - TUMOURS
    - VASCULAR DISEASE
    - SYRINGOBULBIA
    - MOTOR NEURONE DISEASE
    - DIPTHERIA
    - GUILLAIN-BARRE Sy
  - SYMPTOMS
    - DYSARTHRIA
    - DYSPHAGIA
    - NASAL REGURGITATION
  - SIGNS
    - VOCAL CORDS
    - TONGUE
    - STERNOMASTOID / TRAPEZIUS
    - WEAKNESS
    - 11TH Nv
    - PARALYSIS
    - 10TH Nv
    - 12TH Nv
    - 9TH Nv
    - FIBRILLATION
    - WASTING
    - LOSS
    - POSTERIOR 1/3
    - SENSATION
    - TASTE
    - GLOMUS JUGULARE
    - MENINGIOMA
    - NASOPHARYNGEAL
    - JUGULAR FORAMEN

PSEUDOBULBAR PALSY

- CLINICAL
  - CAUSES
    - GENERAL
      - UMN
      - BILATERAL
      - ESSENTIAL
    - VASCULAR
      - HYPERTENSION
    - MS
    - MOTOR NEURONE DISEASE
  - SYMPTOMS
    - SIGNS
      - TONGUE
      - JAW JERK
      - BRISK
      - SLOW MOVING
      - SPASTIC
      - EXTENSOR
      - PLANTAR RESPONSE
      - EMOTIONAL LIABILITY
    - DYSARTHRIA
    - DYSPHAGIA

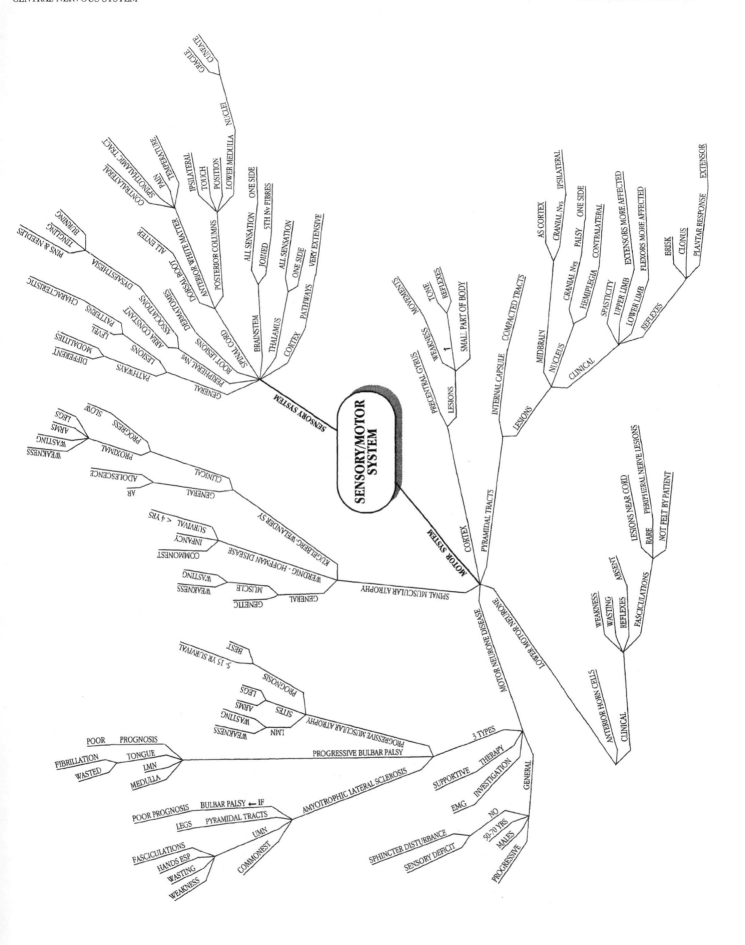

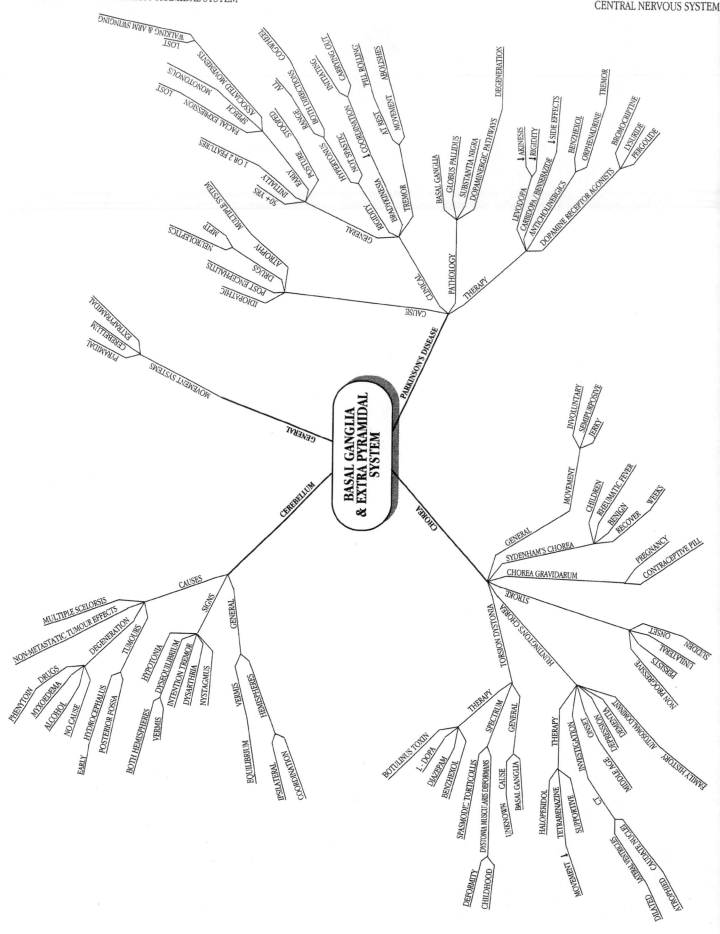

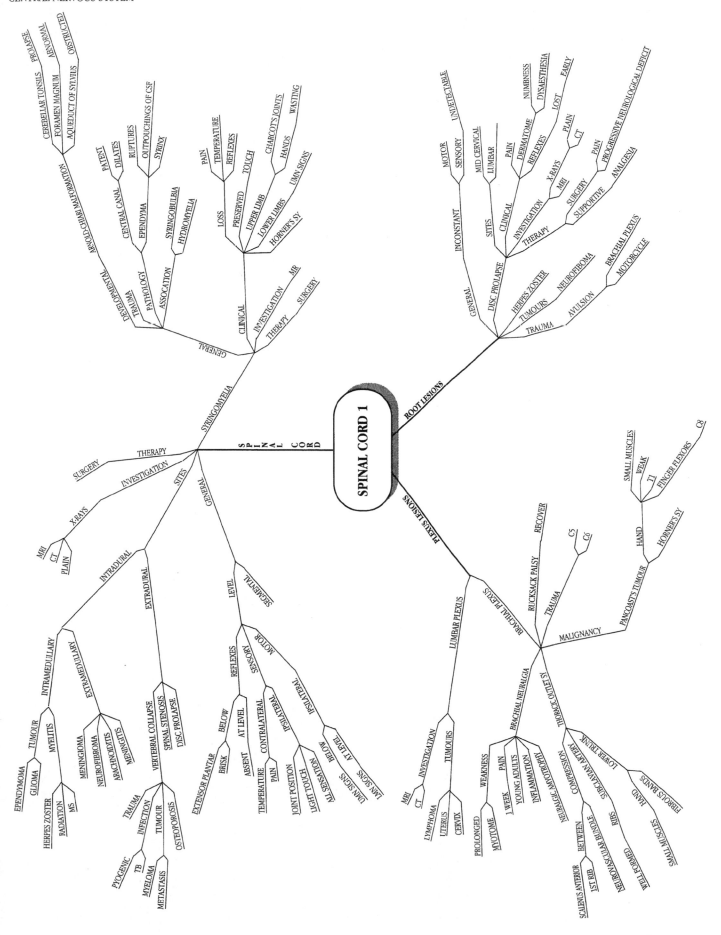

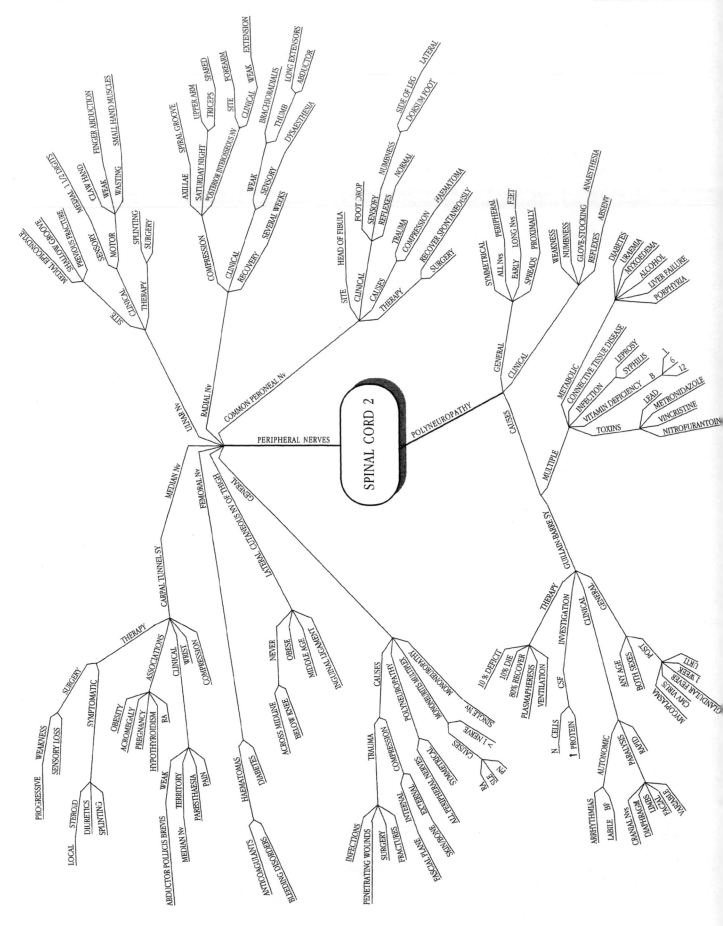

SPINAL CORD 2

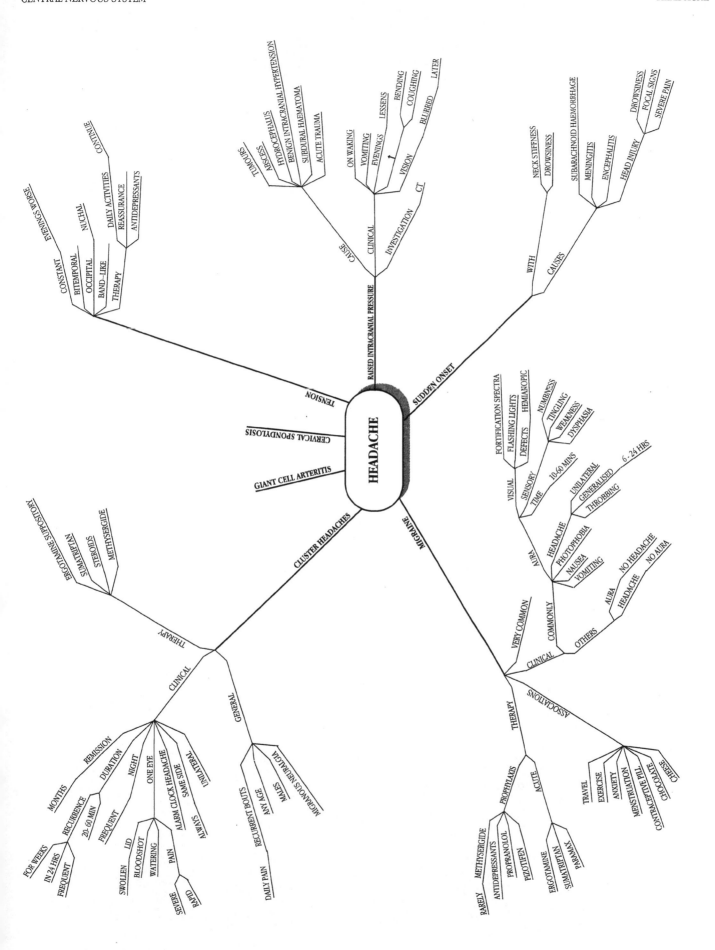

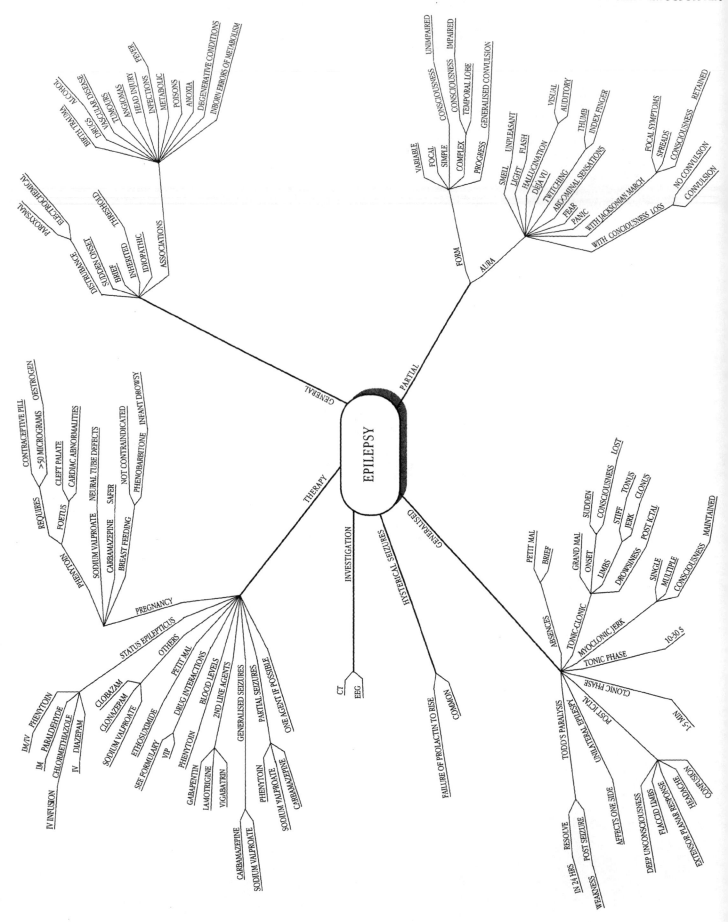

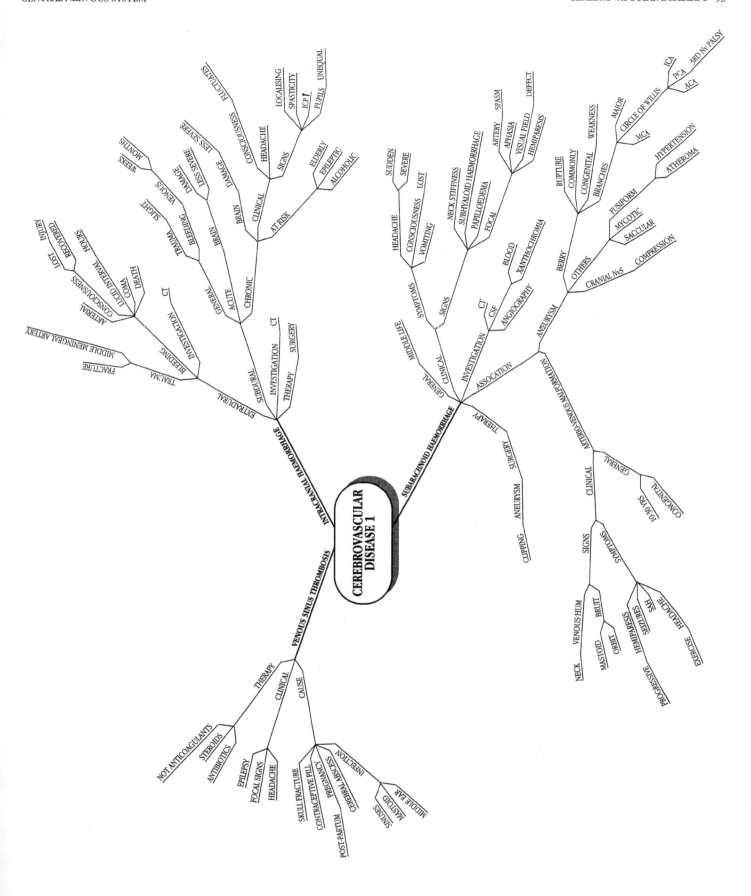

CEREBROVASCULAR DISEASE 1

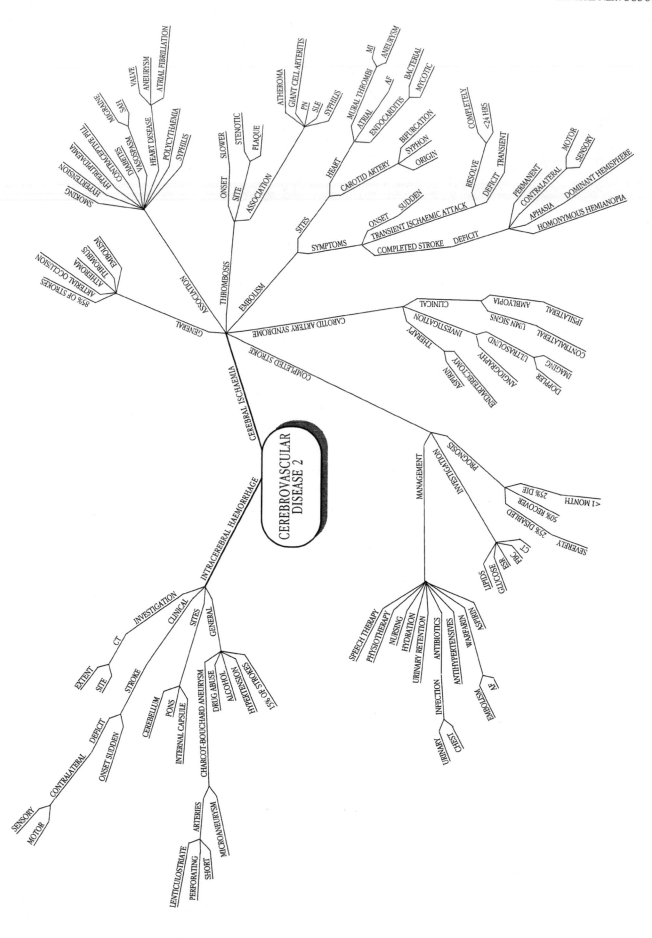

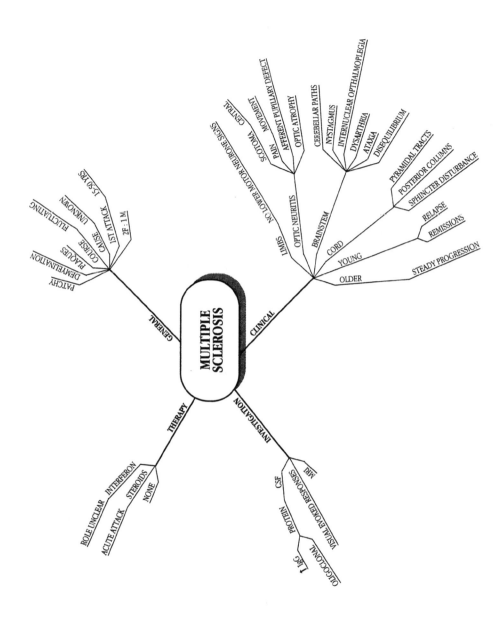

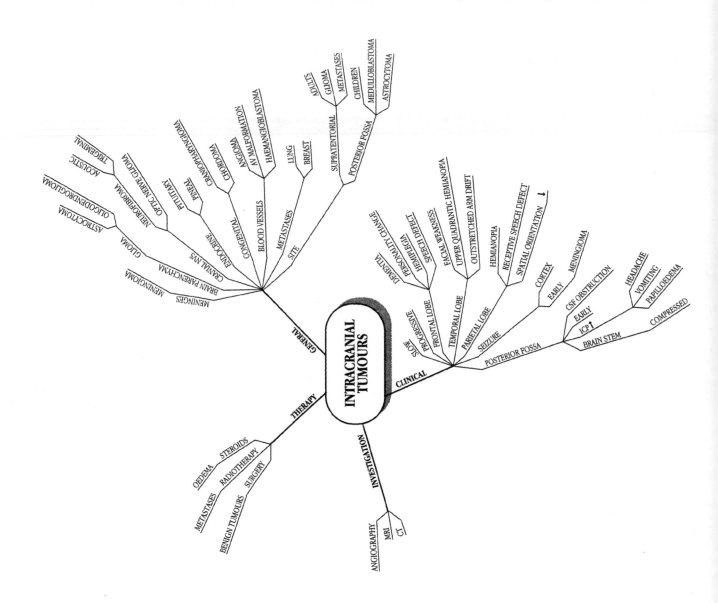

CNS INFECTIONS

VIRAL

AIDS
- PERIPHERAL NEUROPATHY
- ENCEPHALOPATHY — WIDE
- OPPORTUNISTIC — INFECTION — ABSCESS — ATYPICAL — PROGRESSIVE — LATE
- RANGE — PRESENTATION — DEMENTIA — ATAXIA — PYRAMIDAL TRACT SIGNS

CHRONIC VIRAL ENCEPHALITIS
- PROGRESSIVE MULTIFOCAL LEUKOENCEPHALOPATHY
  - PAPOVAVIRUS
  - IMMUNOSUPPRESSION
  - DEMYELINATION — WHITE MATTER — FOCAL — FOCAL SIGNS
  - PROGRESSIVE — DEMENTIA
  - FATAL — MONTHS
- SUBACUTE SCLEROSING PANENCEPHALITIS
  - CLINICAL — RETINITIS — SEIZURES — MYOCLONIC SPASMS — DEMENTIA — YEARS — MONTHS
  - INCUBATION — MEASLES VIRUS
  - CSF — RISING ANTIBODY TITRE
  - DEATH
- JAKOB-CREUTZFELD DISEASE
  - PRION
  - HUMAN TRANSMISSION
  - INCUBATION — YEARS
  - SUBACUTE
  - DEMENTIA
  - SIGNS — EXTRAPYRAMIDAL — MYOCLONUS
  - SEIZURES
  - FATAL — 6 MONTHS

ACUTE VIRAL ENCEPHALITIS
- RABIES
  - HYDROPHOBIA — DRINKING
  - BRAIN — NERVE TRUNKS — 2 MONTHS
  - PRECIPITATE — PHARYNGEAL SPASM — VIRUS TRAVELS — DOG BITES
  - THERAPY — DIPLOID VACCINE — POST INFECTION — GOOD
  - GENERAL — PARALYSIS — RESPIRATORY MUSCLES — DEATH — RAPID — UNCOMMON — FATAL
- POLIOMYELITIS
  - GENERAL — 2 WEEKS — INCUBATION — FLU-LIKE ILLNESS — NASOPHARYNX
- HERPES SIMPLEX
  - INVESTIGATION
    - ANTIBODY TITRE
    - CSF — LYMPHOCYTOSIS — PROTEIN ↑
    - EEG — ABNORMAL
    - CT — ATTENUATION REDUCED — TEMPORAL LOBE — NECROTISING — TEMPORAL LOBE
  - CLINICAL
    - PROGNOSIS — DYSPHASIA — MEMORY DEFICIT — POOR
    - THERAPY — BETAMETHASONE — ACYCLOVIR
    - PROGRESSION — RAPID
    - SEIZURES
    - GENERAL — MOVEMENTS — ABNORMAL — HALLUCINATIONS — DROWSINESS — CONFUSION — ONSET — SUBACUTE — ACUTE — BASAL GANGLIA
  - GENERAL — VIRUSES — RNA — DNA

ACUTE VIRAL MENINGITIS
- GENERAL
- PROGNOSIS — GOOD
- THERAPY — SYMPTOMATIC
- INVESTIGATION — CSF — NORMAL GLUCOSE — LYMPHOCYTOSIS — EARLY POLYMORPHS
- CLINICAL — AS ACUTE MENINGITIS
- CAUSES — GLANDULAR FEVER — MUMPS — ECHOVIRUS — COXSACKIE

BACTERIAL

- SEE INFECTIOUS DISEASES

CHRONIC MENINGITIS
- TUBERCULOSIS
  - GENERAL — HAEMATOGENOUS SPREAD — BASAL — GRANULOMATOUS — HYDROCEPHALUS
  - CLINICAL
    - ONSET — INSIDIOUS
    - SYMPTOMS — WEEKS — HEADACHE — VOMITING — DROWSINESS — DELIRIOUS — CONVULSIONS
    - SIGNS — FEVER — LOW GRADE — CHORDIAL TUBERCLES — PAPILLOEDEMA — CRANIAL Nv PALSIES
  - INVESTIGATION — CSF — ↑ PRESSURE — COBWEB CLOT — LYMPHOCYTOSIS — ↑ PROTEIN — SUGAR LOW — ZIEHL-NEILSON — CULTURE — FILM — WEEKS
  - THERAPY — ANTI-TB CHEMOTHERAPY — 18 MONTHS — STEROIDS — CONTROVERSIAL
- CRYPTOCOCCUS
  - CAUSE — NECFORMANS — FUNGUS
  - THERAPY — AMPHOTERICINE B — 5-FLUOROCYTOSINE

ACUTE MENINGITIS

ABSCESS
- CAUSE — MIDDLE EAR INFECTION — SEPTICAEMIA — SKULL FRACTURE
- CLINICAL — ACUTE — CHRONIC — HEADACHE — PAPILLOEDEMA — FEVER — SEIZURES — SIGNS — FOCAL
- INVESTIGATION — BLOOD — LEUKOCYTOSIS — CULTURE — CT
- THERAPY — ANTIBIOTICS — SURGERY
- MENINGITIS — PAPILLOEDEMA — RESOLVES

NEUROSYPHILIS
- SECONDARY SYPHILIS — MENINGO VASCULAR — ENDARTERITIS — GRANULOMATOUS — CORD — TRANSVERSE MYELITIS
- TERTIARY SYPHILIS — BLOOD — CSF — RAISED PROTEIN — IgG — SEROLOGY +VE — LYMPHOCYTOSIS — +VE SEROLOGY
- GENERAL
- TABES DORSALIS
  - THERAPY — PENICILLIN — HERXHEIMER — REACTION — STEROIDS — PREVENTS
  - GENERAL PARALYSIS OF THE INSANE
    - CSF — ABNORMAL
    - CLINICAL — ARGYLL-ROBERTSON PUPILS — OPTIC ATROPHY — PLANTAR RESPONSE — EXTENSOR — PARAPARESIS — SPASTIC — TREMOR — TONGUE — LIPS — HANDS — SEIZURES — DEMENTIA
    - GENERAL — MENINGO ENCEPHALITIS — SPIROCHAETE PRESENT — CHRONIC
  - CLINICAL
    - DEMYELINATION — POSTERIOR — COLUMNS — ROOTS — ROOT ENTRY ZONE
    - PAIN — POSITION — VIBRATION — LIGHT TOUCH
    - LOSS
    - REFLEXES — ABSENT — DEEP TENDON — TRUNK — NOSE — ARMS — LEGS — HYPOALGESIA
    - SKIN — ULCERS
    - PUPILS — ARGYLL-ROBERTSON — NORMAL CONVERGENCE — LIGHT — UNREACTIVE — IRREGULAR — SMALL
    - NEUROPATHIC JOINTS — FEET — GROSS DISORGANISATION — SITES — ANKLE — CALF — THIGH — ANKLES — KNEES — HIPS — SPINE — SHOULDERS
    - INCONTINENCE — RECTUM — BLADDER
    - IMPOTENCE
    - SENSORY
    - ATAXIA
    - PARAESTHESIA
    - PAIN — LIGHTNING

MUSCLE DISEASE

NEUROMUSCULAR JUNCTION

MYASTHENIA GRAVIS

- GENERAL
  - ANTIBODIES
    - STRIATED MUSCLE
    - ACETYLCHOLINE RECEPTOR
  - CLINICAL
    - EFFECTS
    - SYMPTOMS
      - COMMONLY
      - UNUSUAL
      - ONSET — EYES, BULBAR, NECK, LIMB GIRDLE
      - GRADUAL
      - FLUCTUATING
      - DIPLOPIA
      - DYSPHAGIA
      - DYSARTHRIA
      - CHEWING — DIFFICULT
      - WASTING
      - FASCICULATIONS
      - EXERCISE — ARM
      - REST — RECOVERY, RAPID
      - FATIGUE
      - RELIEVES
      - NOT IN
      - SYMPTOMS FOR 3 MINS
      - OCCULAR
      - BULBAR
    - SIGNS
      - NO
  - INVESTIGATIONS
    - EDROPHONIUM IV
    - EMG
    - CXR — THYMOMA
    - SEROLOGY — ACETYLCHOLINE RECEPTOR Ab
  - THERAPY
    - ANTICHOLINESTERASE DRUGS
    - THYMECTOMY — YOUNG
    - STEROIDS
    - PLASMAPHERESIS — EMERGENCY
    - IMMUNOSUPPRESSION

MYASTHENIC SY

- GENERAL
  - LAMBERT EATON SY
  - ACETYLCHOLINE
  - PRE-JUNCTION
  - RELEASE
  - TUMOURS — SMALL-CELL BRONCHIAL CARCINOMA, FAILURE, OVERT TUMOUR — MONTHS, YEARS
  - PRECEDES
- CLINICAL
  - SYMPTOMS
    - POST EXERTION
  - SIGNS
    - WEAKNESS — PROXIMAL, LIMB GIRDLE
    - REFLEXES — DEPRESSED, ABSENT
    - PARASYMPATHETIC — DRY MOUTH, SPHINCTERS DISTURBED, IMPOTENCE
- INVESTIGATIONS
  - EDROPHONIUM TEST — + VE, NO EFFECT
  - ANTICHOLINESTERASE
  - EMG
- THERAPY
  - GUANIDINE HYDROCHLORIDE
  - STEROIDS
  - IMMUNOSUPPRESSION

ACQUIRED

SYSTEMIC DISEASE RELATED

- SARCOIDOSIS
- RA
- PN
- SLE
- SS
- LIMB GIRDLE
- POLYMYALGIA RHEUMATICA
  - PROXIMAL
  - STEROIDS
  - THYROTOXICOSIS
  - MYXOEDEMA
- DIABETIC AMYOTROPHY
  - FEMORAL NV
  - NEUROPATHY

POLYMYOSITIS

- THERAPY
  - STEROIDS
  - IMMUNOSUPRESSION
- INVESTIGATIONS
  - EMG
  - BIOPSY
  - ↑ ESR
  - ↑ CPK
- ASSOCATIONS
  - OCCULT NEOPLASM
  - DERMATOMYOSITIS — YOUNG
  - RAYNAUD'S SY
- CLINICAL
  - COURSE — RELAPSING
  - REFLEXES — PROLONGED, ABSENT
  - PROXIMAL Ms
  - ARTHRALGIA
  - FEVER
  - MALAISE
  - PAIN
  - ALWAYS — NECK EXTENSORS

MUSCULAR DYSTROPHIES

X-LINKED PSEUDOHYPERTROPHIC

- DUCHENNE
  - WEAKNESS — 3 YRS +, PROXIMAL, LEGS, WALKING, STAIRS
  - PSEUDOHYPERTROPHY — CALF, COMMON
  - CHAIRBOUND — 8-10 YRS
  - FATAL — 15 YRS — CARDIORESPIRATORY FAILURE
  - THERAPY — GENETIC SCREENING, SUPPORTIVE
- BECKER
  - 10% OF CASES
  - AS DUCHENNE
  - MORE BENIGN
  - AD — M=F
  - CLINICAL
    - ADOLESCENCE
    - WEAK — FACE, SHOULDER GIRDLE
    - COURSE — VARIES, BENIGN

FASCIO-SCAPULO-HUMERAL
- AD — M=F

LIMB GIRDLE
- AR — M=F
- ONSET 10-20 YRS
- DISABILITY — SEVERE
- POST ONSET — 20 YRS

MITOCHONDRIAL MYOPATHY
- OCULAR — FACIAL, SHOULDER GIRDLE
- TYPE
- EXTERNAL OPTHALMOPLEGIA — PTOSIS
- COURSE — CHRONIC, YEARS
- AD

MYOTONIC SYNDROMES

DYSTROPHIA MYOTONICA

- CLINICAL
  - GENERAL
  - DYSPHAGIA
  - HORMONES — INSULIN — DIABETES, THYROID, IMPAIRED, GONADS
  - ATROPHY
  - CARDIOMYOCPATHY
  - MYOPATHY — DISTAL — FEET, HANDS
  - CATARACT
  - IQ LOW
  - WEAKNESS
  - WASTING — PTOSIS, FACE
  - BALDNESS — FRONTAL
  - ONSET — ADOLESCENCE
  - ANTICIPATION
  - AD
  - STERNOMASTOID M, TEMPORALIS M, MASSETER M
  - MANIFESTATIONS ↓
  - SUCCEEDING GENERATIONS

MYOTONICA CONGENITA

- MUSCLES — LITTLE HERCULES, HYPERTROPHIED
- ONSET — BIRTH
- AD
- THOMSENS DISEASE

MISCELLANEOUS CNS

NEUROFIBROMATOSIS

- GENERAL
  - CLINICAL
    - AUTOSOMAL DOMINANT
    - NERVOUS SYSTEM
      - SKIN
        - PATCHY
        - CAFÉ AU LAIT SPOTS — >5
      - RETINA
        - PHACOMAS
      - SKELETON
        - BONY MODELLING
          - SKULL
          - SPINE
        - ABNORMAL
          - THICKENING
          - KYPHOSCOLIOSIS
      - CRANIAL NVS
        - PIGMENTATION
        - NODULES
          - Type I
          - Type II
          - PERIPHERAL
          - CENTRAL
      - SPINAL ROOTS
        - ESPECIALLY 5, 8, 9
        - DUMBBELL
        - CORD COMPRESSION
  - COMPLICATIONS
    - GLIOMA
    - EPENDYMOMA
    - MENINGIOMA
    - SARCOMA
    - ARACHNOID CYSTS

DEFICIENCY STATES

- VITAMIN B1
  - BERI-BERI
    - PERIPHERAL NVS
      - HANDS & FEET
        - PAIN
        - PARAESTHESIA
        - WEAKNESS
        - WASTING
        - REFLEXES — ABSENT
        - SENSORY LOSS
          - GLOVE
          - STOCKING
    - WET BERI BERI
      - CARDIAC FAILURE
  - KORSAKOFF'S PSYCHOSIS
    - POLYNEURITIS
    - CONFUSION
    - DISORIENTATION
    - MEMORY LOSS — RECENT
    - CONFABULATION
  - WERNICKE'S ENCEPHALOPATHY
    - ASSOCIATION
      - KORSAKOFF'S PSYCHOSIS
      - POLYNEURITIS
    - CLINICAL
      - CONFUSION
      - DROWSINESS
      - NYSTAGMUS
      - OCULAR PALSIES
      - ATAXIA — TRUNCAL
- VITAMIN B12
  - MACROCYTIC ANAEMIA
  - SUBACUTE COMBINED DEGENERATION OF CORD
    - SITES
      - POSTERIOR COLUMNS
      - LATERAL COLUMNS
    - THERAPY
      - HYDROXYCOBALAMIN
      - LIFE LONG
    - CLINICAL
      - SIGNS
        - OPTIC ATROPHY
        - DEMENTIA
        - REFLEXES
          - PLANTAR RESPONSES — EXTENSOR
          - ABSENT — ANKLE, KNEE
      - SYMPTOMS
        - SENSORY ATAXIA
        - PARAESTHESIA — FEET, HANDS
        - PYRAMIDAL TRACTS — LEGS, 1ST AFFECTED
        - IMPAIRED
          - JOINT POSITION
          - VIBRATION
          - TOUCH

HEREDITARY SPINOCEREBELLAR DEGENERATIONS

- PERONEAL MUSCULAR ATROPHY · CHARCOT - MARIE - TOOTH DISEASE
  - TYPES
    - 1 — AD, DEMYELINATION, 1ST DECADE ONSET
    - 2 — AD, AXONAL, 5TH DECADE ONSET
  - PERIPHERAL NVS
    - CLINICAL
      - MUSCLE
        - PES CAVUS
        - WEAKNESS
        - WASTING
        - PERONEI
        - MID THIGH — STOPS AT
      - ONSET
- FRIEDREICH'S ATAXIA
  - GENERAL
    - COMMONEST
    - AUTOSOMAL RECESSIVE
    - CHILDREN
  - CLINICAL
    - HEART
      - CARDIOMYOPATHY
    - PES CAVUS
      - ONSET
      - CLUMSY
      - HANDS
      - GAIT
      - UNSTEADY
    - SITES
      - OPTIC Nv
        - PERIPHERAL NVS
          - REFLEXES ABSENT
      - SEVERITY — LESS / MORE
        - WEAK LEGS
        - PYRAMIDAL COLUMNS
          - PLANTAR RESPONSES — EXTENSOR
      - CORD
        - POSTERIOR COLUMNS — ABSENT
          - VIBRATION SENSE
          - PROPRIOCEPTION
      - CEREBELLUM
        - ATAXIA
        - DYSARTHRIA
        - NYSTAGMUS
  - GENERAL
    - PERIPHERAL NVS
    - SPINAL CORD
    - CEREBELLUM

NON METASTATIC SYNDROMES

- MYELOPATHY
- CEREBELLAR ATROPHY
- DEMENTIA
- POLYNEUROPATHY
  - SENSORY
  - MOTOR
- TUMOURS
  - LYMPHOMA
  - MYELOMA
  - LUNG — SMALL CELL

Blood disease

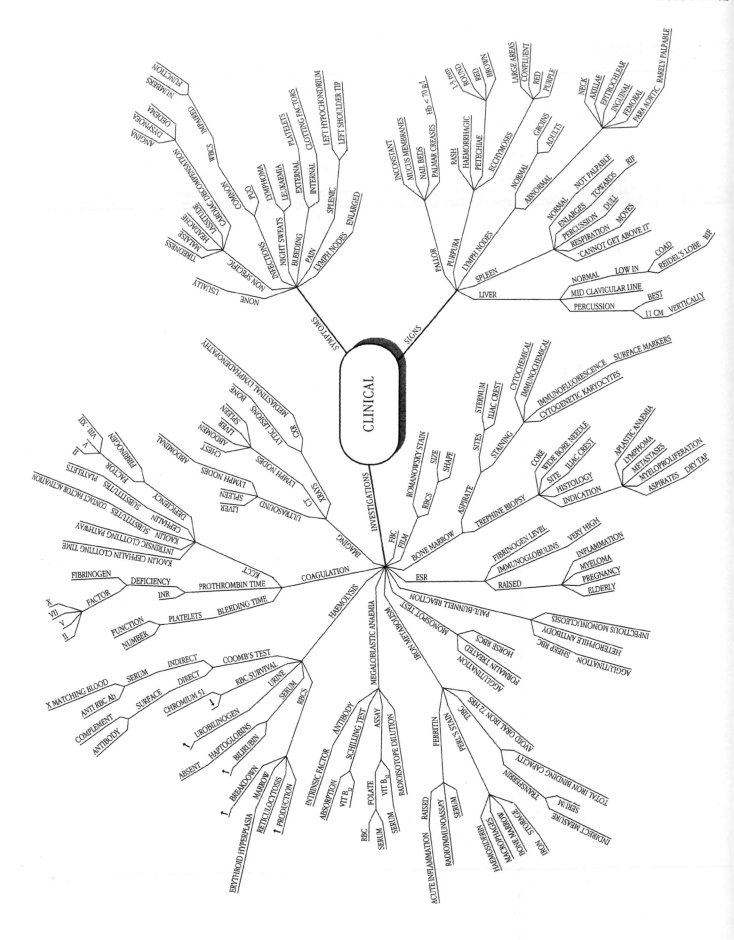

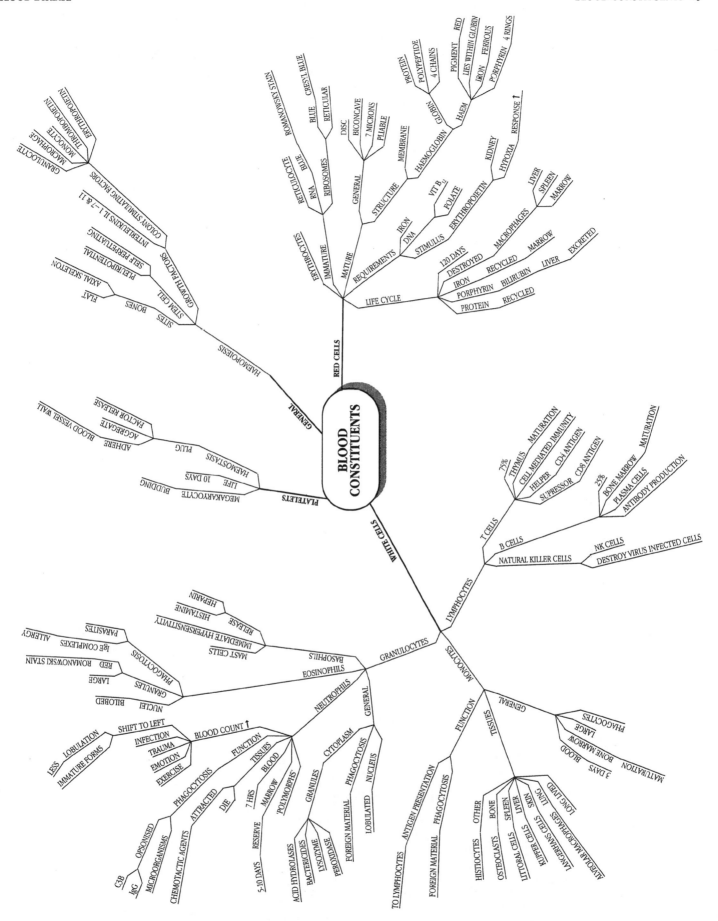

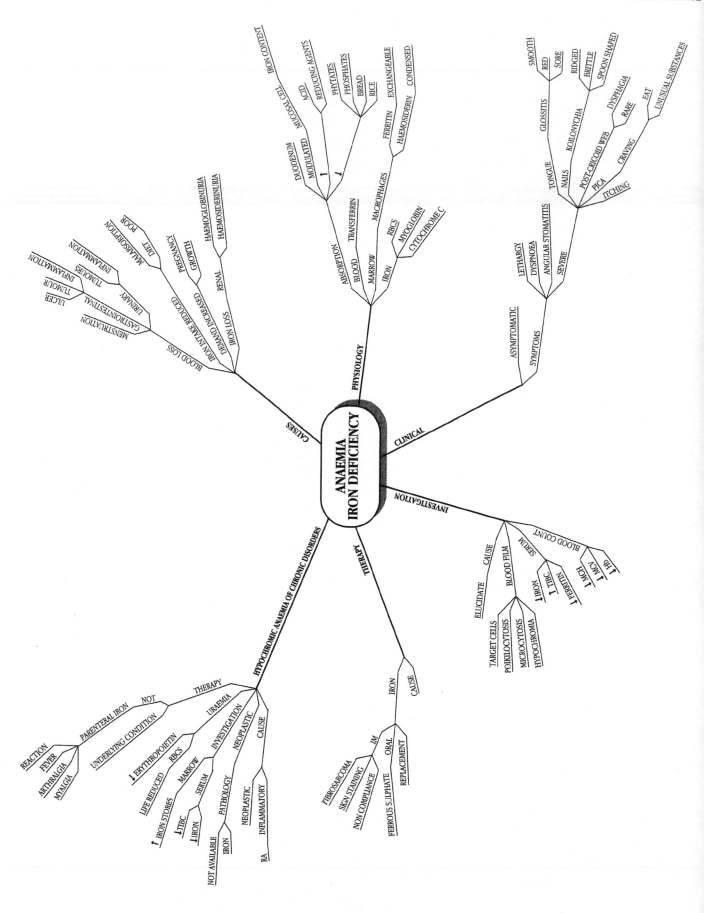

ANAEMIA MEGALOBLASTIC

CAUSE

DEFICIENCY

VIT B$_{12}$
- INTAKE ↓
  - VEGANS
- INTRINSIC FACTOR ↓
  - STOMACH
    - PERNICIOUS ANAEMIA
    - GASTRECTOMY PARTIAL
    - CONGENITAL
  - SMALL INTESTINE
    - BACTERIAL OVERGROWTH
      - STAGNANT LOOP
    - COELIAC DISEASE
    - TROPICAL SPRUE
    - FISH TAPEWORM
    - TERMINAL ILEUM
      - CROHN'S DISEASE
      - RESECTION

FOLATE
- INTAKE ↓
  - MALABSORPTION
    - ALCOHOLICS
    - ELDERLY
    - POVERTY
    - COELIAC DISEASE
    - TROPICAL SPRUE
    - RESECTION
    - BOWEL
  - NEED ↑
    - PREGNANCY
    - LACTATION
    - BLOOD DISEASE
      - HAEMOLYSIS
      - MYELOFIBROSIS
      - LYMPHOMA
      - CARCINOMA
    - NEOPLASM
    - INFLAMMATION
      - SKIN
        - EXFOLIATION
      - RA
      - ICU
    - DRUGS
      - PATIENTS
      - PHENYTOIN
      - ANTIFOLATES
        - METHOTREXATE

RESISTANCE
- CONGENITAL
  - LESCH-NYHAN SY
  - OROTIC ACIDURIA
- METABOLIC INHIBITORS
  - 6 MERCAPTOURINE
  - 6 THIOGUANINE
  - 5 FLUOOURACIL
  - HYDROXYURIA
  - CYTOSINE ARABINOSIDE

PHYSIOLOGY

VIT B$_{12}$
- COMPOUND
  - COBALT
- PRODUCE
  - BACTERIA
  - NOT VEGETABLES
- STOMACH
  - RELEASED VIT B$_{12}$
  - INTRINSIC FACTOR
    - BINDING
    - GLYCOPROTEIN
    - PORTAL BLOOD
- TERMINAL ILEUM
  - ABSORBED
- PORTAL BLOOD
  - TRANSCOBALAMIN 2
- BONE MARROW
- STORAGE
  - LIVER
  - 4 YEARS

FOLATE
- VEGETABLES
- YEAST
- POLYGLUTAMATES
- METHYL TETRAHYDROFOLATE
  - PLASMA
  - CELL UPTAKE
    - VIT B$_{12}$
    - THYMIDINE
  - COENZYME
  - DNA
  - PRODUCTION

GENERAL

RBC
- MATURATION
  - NUCLEUS
    - DELAYED
  - DNA
    - DEFECT
  - CYTOPLASM
    - NORMAL
  - IN SYNTHESIS

THERAPY

RESPONSE
- RETICULOCYTOSIS
- POTASSIUM SUPPLEMENTS
  - ELDERLY
- FOLIC ACID
- VIT B$_{12}$
  - HYDROXYCOBALAMIN

INVESTIGATION

FOLATE
- SERUM
  - FOLATE ↓
- BLOOD
  - RED CELL FOLATE ↓
  - MACROCYTOSIS

VIT B$_{12}$
- BONE MARROW
  - SCHILLING TEST
    - UNRESPONSIVE TO VIT B$_{12}$
- BLOOD
  - NEUTROPHILS
    - HYPERSEGMENTED
  - MACROCYTOSIS
  - <150 pg/ml
- SERUM
  - ANTIBODIES
    - INTRINSIC FACTOR
    - PARIETAL CELLS

COMPLICATIONS

NEUROLOGICAL
- OPTIC ATROPHY
- DEMENTIA
- PERIPHERAL NEUROPATHY
  - VERY RARE
  - GLOVE - STOCKING
- SUBACUTE COMBINED DEGENERATION OF CORD

PERNICIOUS ANAEMIA

CLINICAL
- STOMACH
  - CARCINOMA
- INFERTILITY
  - FEMALES
- SPLENOMEGALY
- PURPURA
- JAUNDICE
- MILD
- GLOSSITIS
- INSIDIOUS ONSET

GENERAL
- GASTRIC MUCOSA
  - PARIETAL CELLS
  - ATROPHIC
  - ACID REDUCED
- ANTIBODIES
- AUTOIMMUNE DISEASE

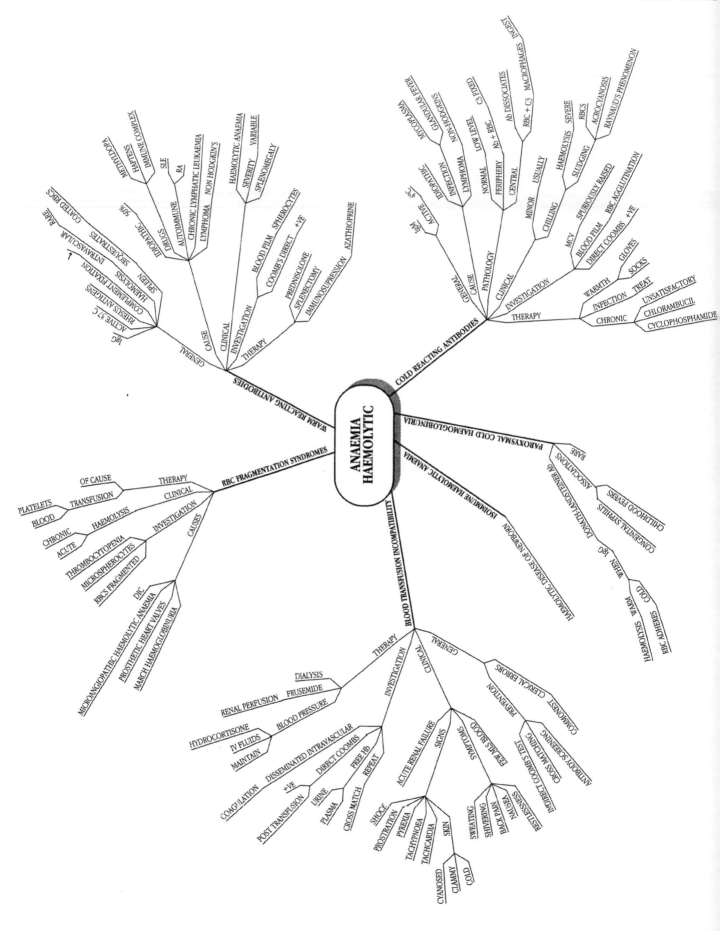

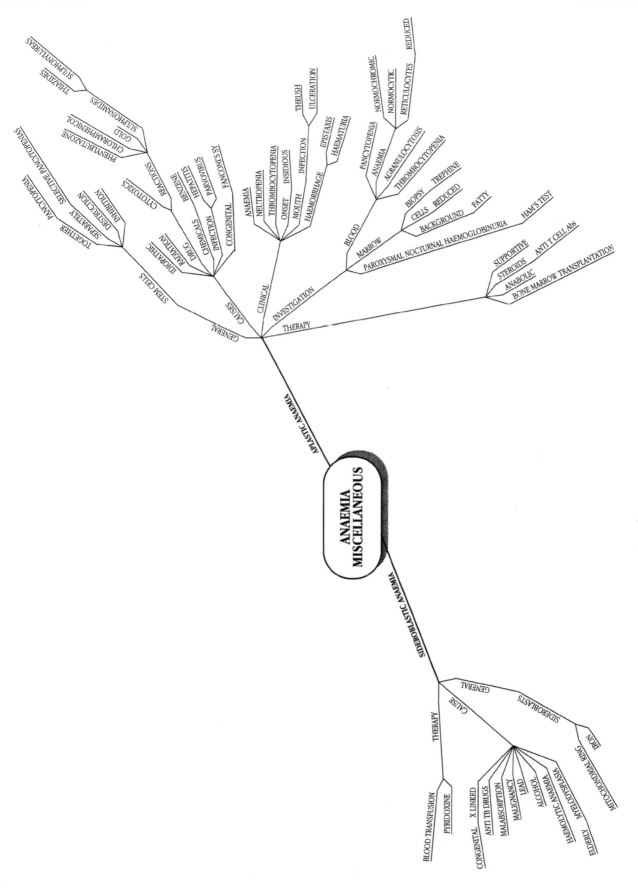

ANAEMIA MISCELLANEOUS

APLASTIC ANAEMIA

GENERAL

STEM CELLS

CAUSES

IDIOPATHIC

RADIATION

DRUG

CHEMICALS

INFECTION

CONGENITAL

REACTIONS

CYTOTOXICS

BENZENE

HEPATITIS

PARVOVIRUS

FANCONI'S SY

PHENYLBUTAZONE

CHLORAMPHENICOL

GOLD

SULPHONAMIDES

THIAZIDES

SULPHONYLUREAS

SEPARATELY

TOGETHER

PANCYTOPENIA

SELECTIVE PANCYTOPENIA

DESTRUCTION

INHIBITION

CLINICAL

ANAEMIA

NEUTROPENIA

THROMBOCYTOPENIA

ONSET

INSIDIOUS

MOUTH

INFECTION

HAEMORRHAGE

EPISTAXIS

HAEMATURIA

THRUSH

ULCERATION

INVESTIGATION

BLOOD

PANCYTOPENIA

ANAEMIA

AGRANULOCYTOSIS

THROMBOCYTOPENIA

NORMOCHROMIC

NORMOCYTIC

RETICULOCYTES

REDUCED

MARROW

BIOPSY

TREPHINE

CELLS

REDUCED

BACKGROUND

FATTY

PAROXYSMAL NOCTURNAL HAEMOGLOBINURIA

HAM'S TEST

THERAPY

SUPPORTIVE

STEROIDS

ANABOLIC

ANTI T CELL Abs

BONE MARROW TRANSPLANTATION

SIDEROBLASTIC ANAEMIA

GENERAL

SIDEROBLASTS

IRON

MITOCHONDRIAL RING

CAUSE

CONGENITAL

X LINKED

ANTI TB DRUGS

MALABSORPTION

MALIGNANCY

LEAD

ALCOHOL

HAEMOLYTIC ANAEMIA

MYELODYSPLASIA

ELDERLY

THERAPY

BLOOD TRANSFUSION

PYRIDOXINE

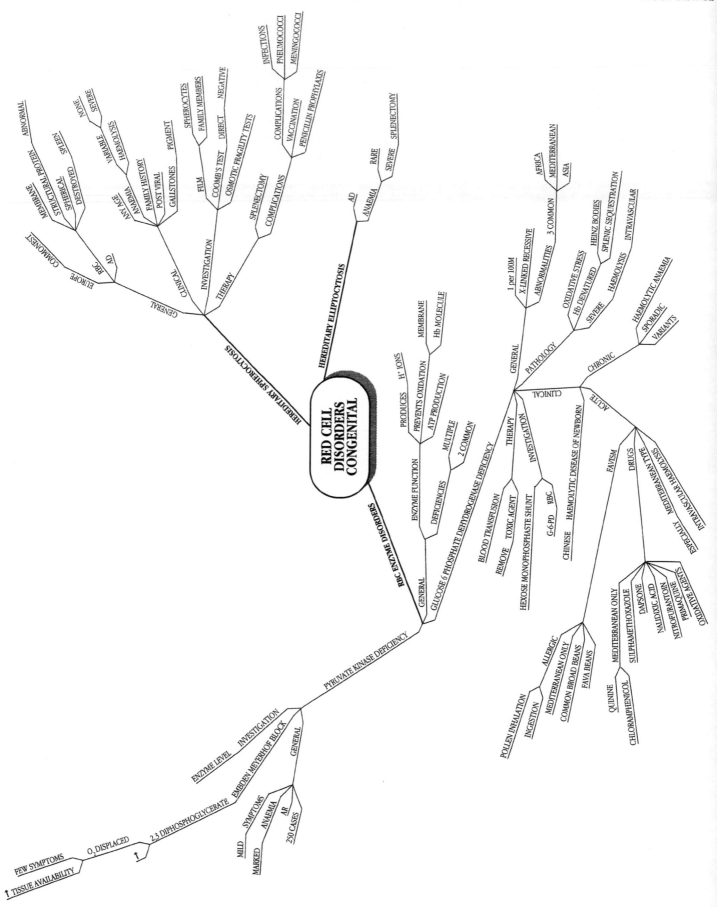

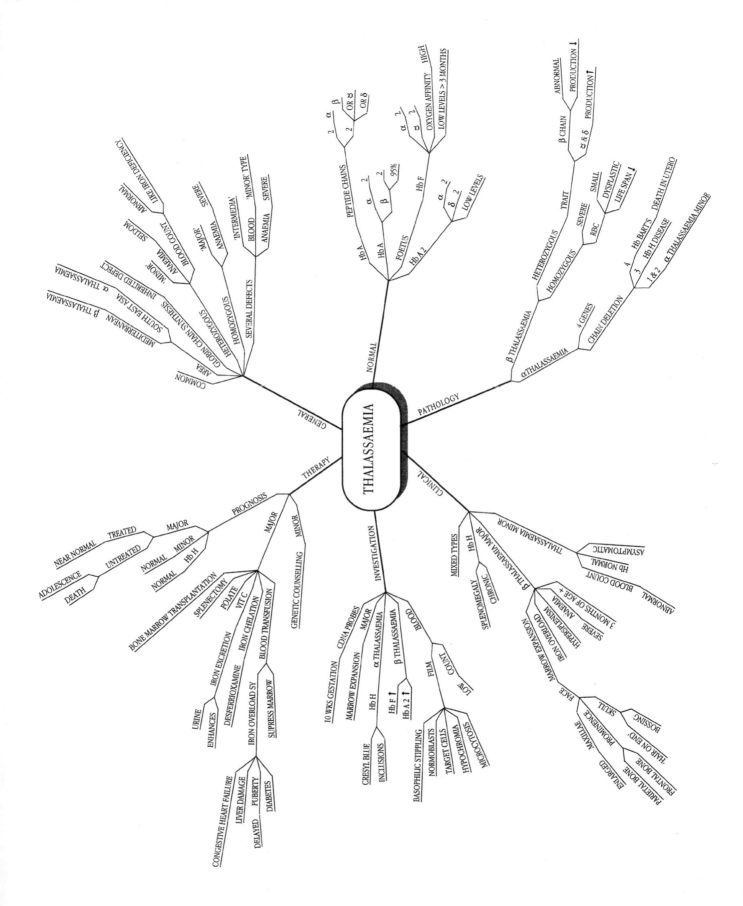

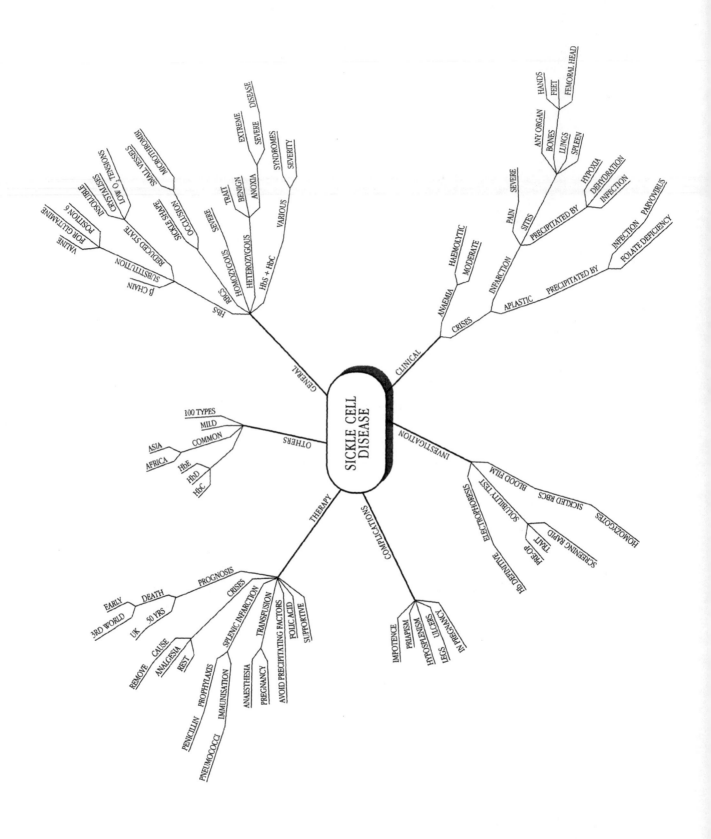

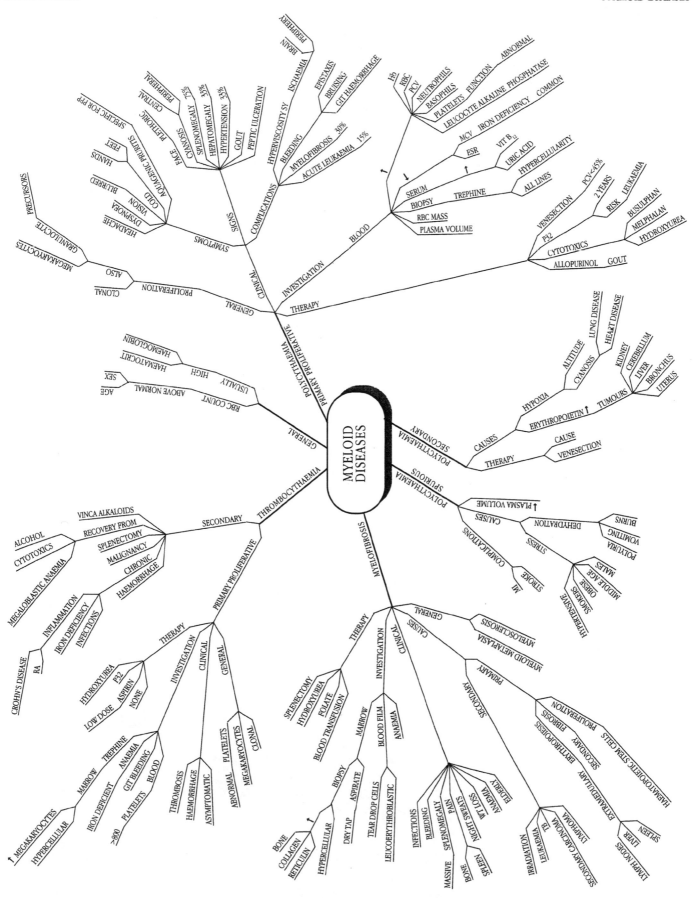

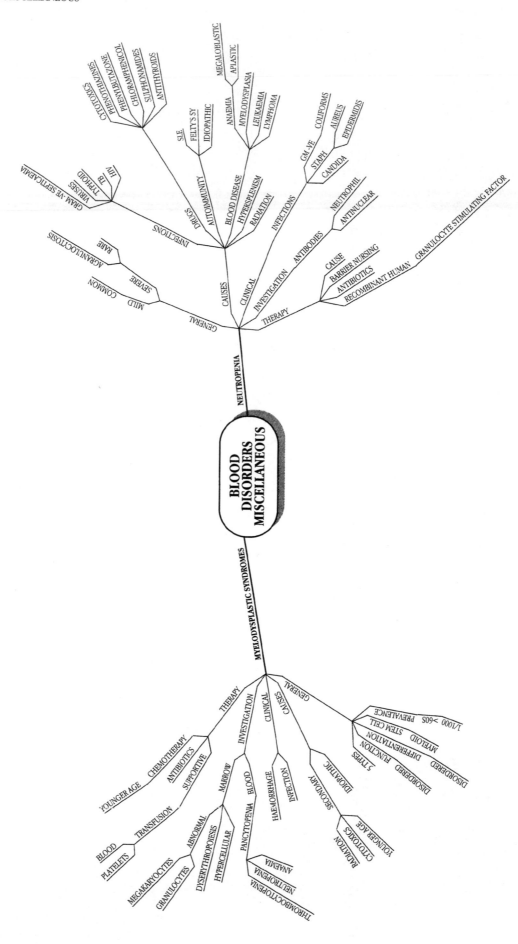

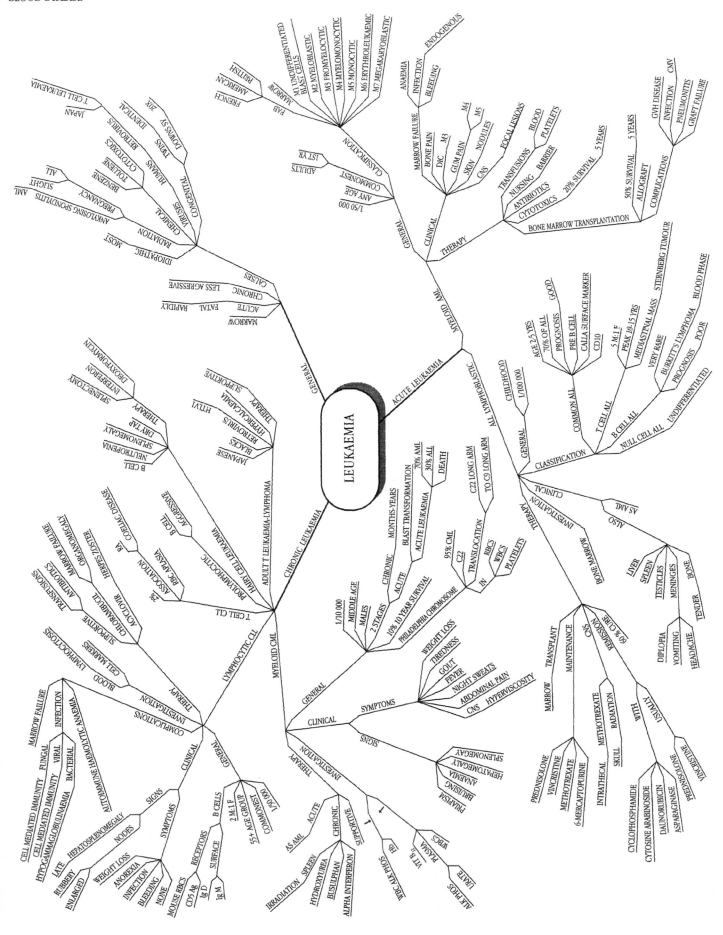

LEUKAEMIA

LYMPHOMA

HODGKIN'S DISEASE

GENERAL

CLINICAL

- SYMPTOMS
  - LYMPHADENOPATHY — PAINLESS, MARKED, SITES (NECK, AXILLA, GROIN)
  - FEVER
  - WEIGHT LOSS
  - NIGHT SWEATS
  - PRURITIS
  - TIREDNESS
  - PEL-EBSTEIN FEVER — ALTERNATE (FEVER, LOW TEMP, 2-4 WEEKS), ALSO IN (TB)
- SIGNS
  - NODES — ENLARGED
  - ORGANOMEGALY — LIVER, SPLEEN, MARROW — RENAL CARCINOMA

INVESTIGATION

- BIOPSY
- BLOOD — ANAEMIA, NEUTROPENIA, EOSINOPHILIA
- CT — CHEST, ABDOMEN

STAGING

- PROGNOSIS — 1, 2, 3, 4
- SINGLE REGION
- DIAPHRAGM — SAME SIDE, BOTH SIDES, > 1 REGION
- EXTRANODAL SPREAD
- SYMPTOMLESS
- A SYMPTOMS
- B SYMPTOMS

THERAPY

- IRRADIATION — 1 TO 2A
- CHEMOTHERAPY — 2B TO 4B
- PROGNOSIS — 80% 5YR SURVIVAL

SPREAD

- CLASSIFICATION
  - REED-STERNBERG CELLS — BINUCLEATE, MIRROR IMAGE
  - LYMPHOCYTE PREDOMINANT
  - NODULAR SCLEROSING
  - MIXED CELLULARITY
  - LYMPHOCYTE DEPLETED
  - NODAL

NON-HODGKIN'S LYMPHOMA

GENERAL

MALIGNANCY

- LOW-GRADE (35%)
  - LYMPHOCYTES, CENTROCYTES, IMMUNOCYTES
  - SMALLER CELLS
  - HISTOLOGY — NODULAR
  - COURSE — PROLONGED
  - SURVIVAL — GOOD
  - SPARES — TESTES, BRAIN
  - CHEMOTHERAPY — GOOD RESPONSE, NO CURE
- INTERMEDIATE (20%) — T CELL ORIGIN, HIGH-GRADE
- HIGH-GRADE
  - MISCELLANEOUS — UNCLASSIFIED, HISTIOCYTIC LYMPHOMA (T CELLS), MYCOSIS FUNGOIDES
    - CHEMOTHERAPY — MISCELLANEOUS, MAY CURE
    - SPARES — NOTHING
    - COURSE — SHORT
    - HISTOLOGY — DIFFUSE, LARGER CELLS, 35%

CLINICAL

- LYMPH NODES — 60% > 50YRS
- HEPATOSPLENOMEGALY
- EXTRANODAL — BONE, THYROID, LUNG, STOMACH, SKIN
- DISSEMINATED — 85%
- RETROPERITONEUM — 10%
- OROPHARYNGEAL
- SUPERFICIAL
- PAINLESS
- ASYMMETRIC
- ENLARGED

INVESTIGATION — CT, US, CXR, BIOPSY

THERAPY

- HIGH GRADE — MARROW TRANSPLANT
  - < 2 YEARS
  - DEATH — 30%
  - CURE
  - RELAPSE — FREQUENT
  - RESPONSE — GOOD
  - CHEMOTHERAPY
- LOW GRADE
  - SURVIVAL — 7 YEARS
  - AGGRESSIVE
  - TRANSFORMS
  - RADIOTHERAPY — LOCALISED
  - CHEMOTHERAPY — SINGLE AGENT
  - NONE

BURKITT'S LYMPHOMA

GENERAL

- B CELL
- LYMPHOBLASTIC
- AREA — MALARIAL REGIONS (NEW GUINEA, AFRICA)
- YOUNG
- EB VIRUS
- CHROMOSOMAL TRANSLOCATION
- AIDS

CLINICAL

- SITES — BREAST, OVARIES, ADRENALS, KIDNEYS, JAW, EXTRANODAL

INVESTIGATION

- BIOPSY — STARRY SKY, SHEETS, LYMPHOID CELLS, HISTIOCYTES

THERAPY

- DIFFUSE — B CELL LYMPHOBLASTIC
- LOCALISED
- PROGNOSIS — POOR
- CHEMOTHERAPY — CYCLOPHOSPHAMIDE

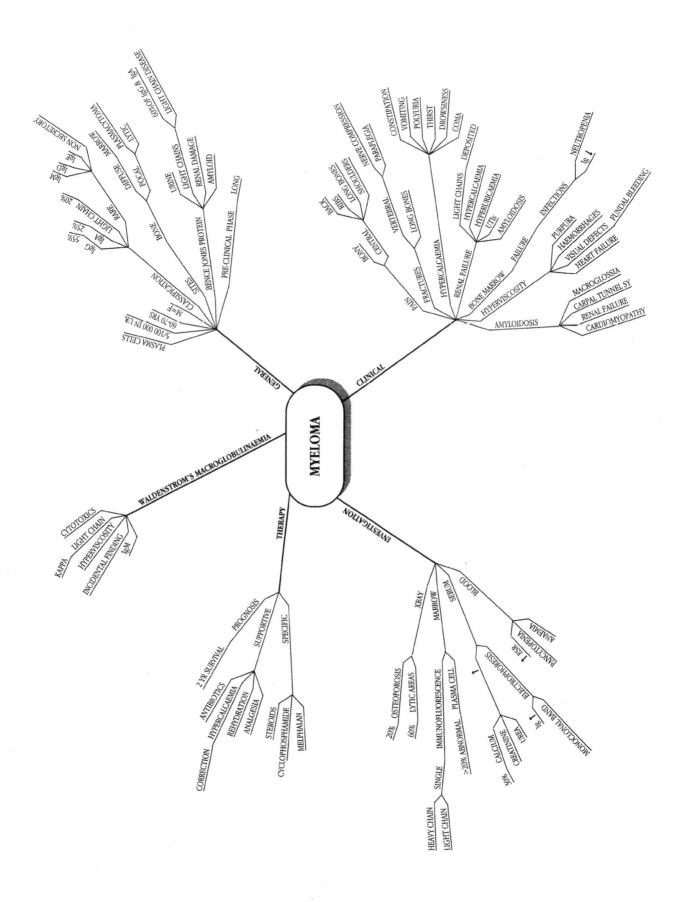

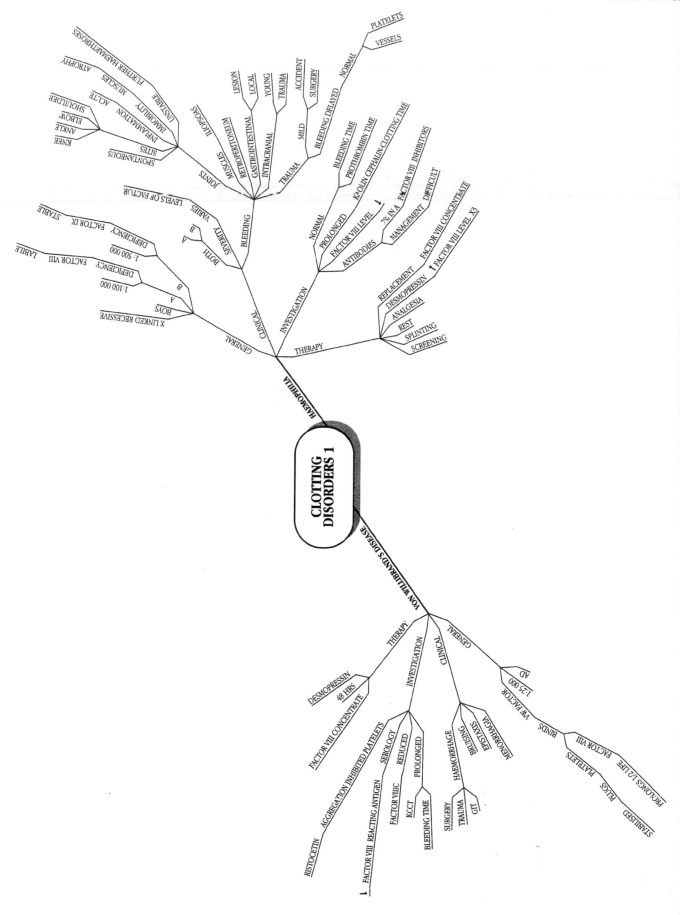

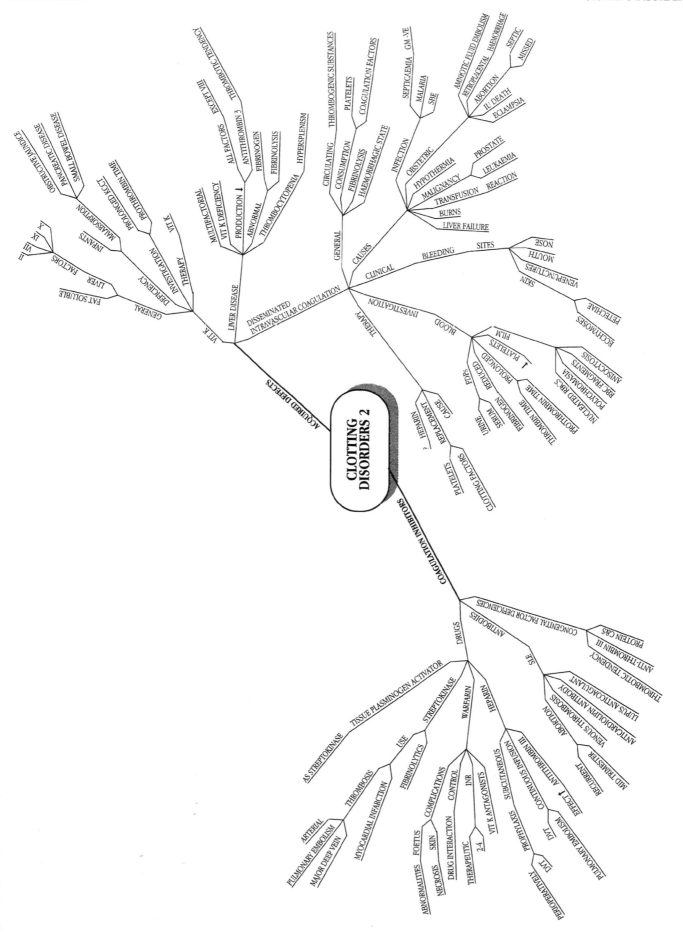

CLOTTING DISORDERS 2

Kidney

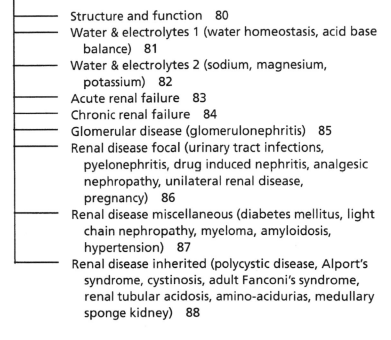

STRUCTURE AND FUNCTION

STRUCTURE

NEPHRON

CORTEX
- CAPILLARY — NETWORK, ENDOTHELIUM, AFFERENT IN, EFFERENT OUT
- BASEMENT MEMBRANE
- EPITHELIUM
- MESANGIUM

GLOMERULUS
- CAPILLARY
  - BASEMENT MEMBRANE — 3 LAYERS, −VE CHARGE, FUSE, PROTEINURIA
  - GBM
  - FOOT PROCESSES
- EPITHELIUM — OUTER LAYER, CELLS, PHAGOCYTES, SECRETED BY, CELLS
- MESANGIUM — MATRIX, GBM, PRODUCTION

PROXIMAL CONVOLUTED TUBULE
- PCT
- CORTEX
- LUMEN
- REABSORPTION
- MEDULLA
- CONCENTRATION OF URINE
- ACTIVE TRANSPORT
- COUNTERCURRENT MECHANISMS
- LH — PATENT, NORMAL, COLLAPSE, ISCHAEMIA, GLOMERULAR FILTRATE

LOOP OF HENLE
- DCT, CORTEX
- ACTIVE TRANSPORT
- NaCl
- IMPERMEABLE TO WATER
- SECRETION, K+

DISTAL CONVOLUTED TUBULE
- CD
- MEDULLA
- SECRETION — H+, K+, NH3
- REABSORPTION, BICARBONATE

COLLECTING DUCTS

INTERSTITIUM
- MATRIX
- CELLS
- FUNCTION — STRUCTURAL, SUPPORT, HLA, EXPRESSION, PROSTAGLANDIN, SECRETION

FUNCTION

GENERAL
- 20% CARDIAC OUTPUT
  - ULTRAFILTRATE — GLOMERULUS, DIFFUSION, PASSIVE
  - REABSORPTION — TUBULES, SELECTIVE
  - EXCRETION — TUBULES, ACTIVE
  - ENDOCRINE
    - ERYTHROPOIETIN — RBC PRODUCTION, CRF ↓, ANAEMIA, RENAL CYSTIC DISEASE, PRODUCTION
    - RENIN — ENZYME, JUXTAGLOMERULAR APPARATUS, FUNCTION, ANGIOTENSIN 1, ALDOSTERONE RELEASE, BLOOD, PRESSURE, VOLUME
    - 1,25 DIHYDROXYCHOLECALCIFEROL — CONTROLS, CALCIUM ABSORPTION, RENAL FAILURE, ↓ CALCIUM ABSORPTION, ↓ SKELETAL GROWTH, RENAL OSTEODYSTROPHY

- CAUSES — EXERCISE, FEVERS, HEART FAILURE, GLOMERULONEPHRITIS, INTERSTITIAL NEPHRITIS, PREGNANCY, NEPHROTIC SY

PROTEINURIA
- INFECTION
- GN
- PROSTATIC HYPERTROPHY, KIDNEY, URINARY TRACT
- TUMOURS
- RENAL CYSTIC DISEASE
- PAPILLARY NECROSIS
- BLEEDING DISORDERS

HAEMATURIA

PYURIA — CALCULI, INFECTION, ANALGESIC NEPHROPATHY, CYSTITIS, INTERSTITIAL NEPHRITIS, TUBULO-INTERSTITIAL NEPHRITIS

MICROSCOPY
- ORGANISMS — GN, RBCS DYSMORPHIC
- CASTS
  - FORMED — DCT, CD, TAMM-HORSFALL PROTEIN, CYLINDRICAL, HYALINE
  - NORMAL, EXERCISE, DIURETICS, EPITHELIAL
  - WBC CASTS — ACUTE TUBULAR NECROSIS, PYELONEPHRITIS, GN, PATHOGNOMONIC
  - RBC CASTS

URINE / PLASMA
- UREA — VARIES WITH ↑, GFR < 70%, UNRELIABLE, GI BLEEDING, LIVER FUNCTION, HYDRATION, CATABOLISM, PROTEIN INTAKE, GFR < 50% ↑
- CREATININE — VARIES, PRODUCTION CONSTANT ↑, M > F, MUSCLE MASS, DRUGS, ASPIRIN, COTRIMOXAZOLE, TETRACYCLINE

GFR
- CREATININE CLEARANCE — RADIOISOTOPES, AGENTS, VARIES
- 24 HR URINE COLLECTION — SINGLE BLOOD SAMPLE, UNRELIABLE, TIMED, BLOOD SAMPLES, SINGLE INJECTION
- GROSS OEDEMA
- EXCRETION, REABSORPTION, NO, FREELY FILTERED, GBM PERMEABILITY, FILTRATION PRESSURE

TUBULAR FUNCTION
- PROXIMAL
  - URINE — TUBULAR, PROTEINURIA, GLYCOSURIA, AMINOACIDURIA
  - SERUM — ↓ PO4, ↓ K+
- DISTAL
  - RENAL ACIDOSIS — URINE pH > 5.3, DCT, NOT SECRETED, H+, HCO3−, ↓ REABSORPTION, LOST, NORMALISES, DESMOPRESSIN
  - OSMOLALITY — FLUID DEPRIVATION TEST, DIABETES INSIPIDUS, REPEAT OSMOLALITY, OVERNIGHT, EARLY MORNING URINE, NORMAL > 550 mOsmol/kg

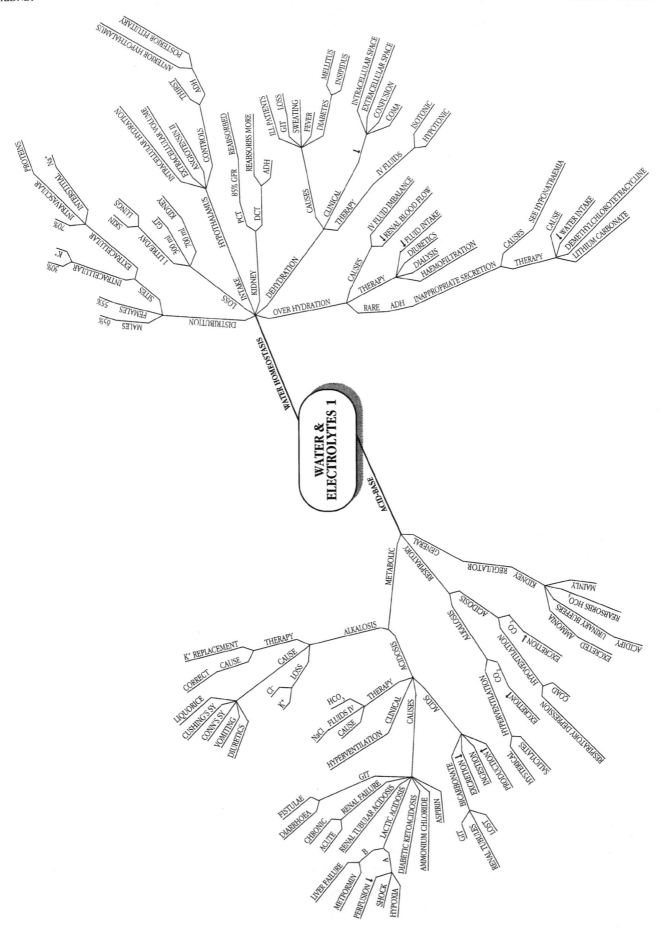

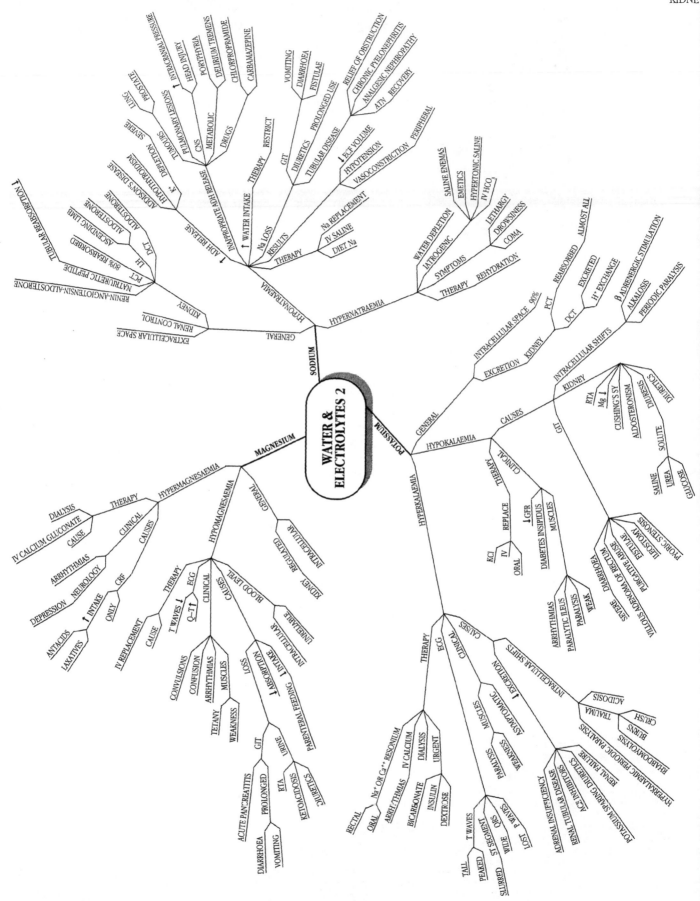

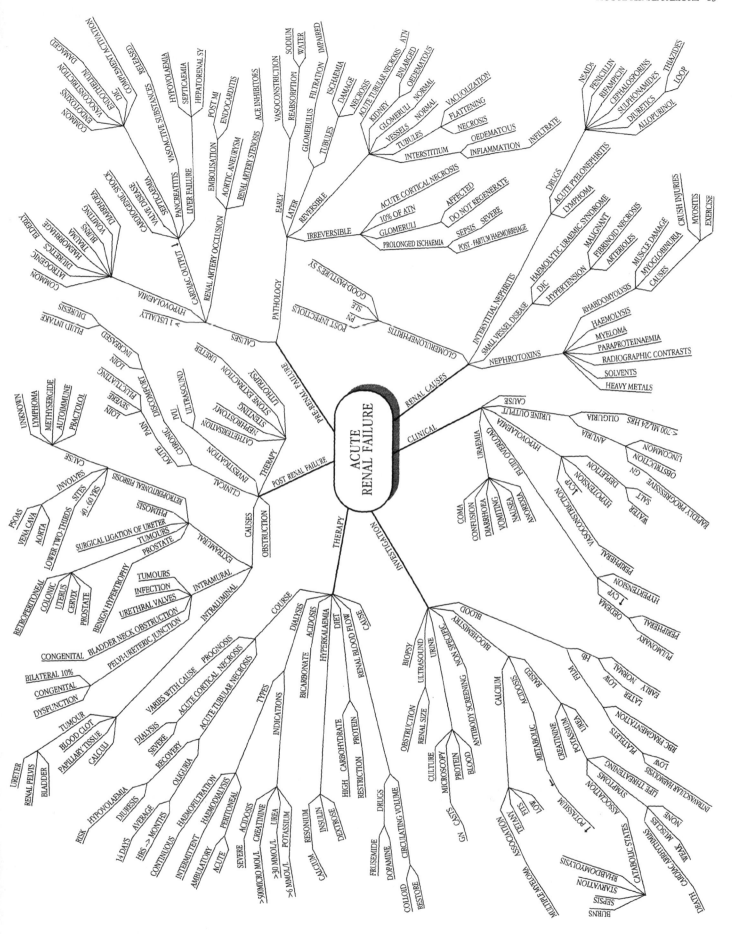

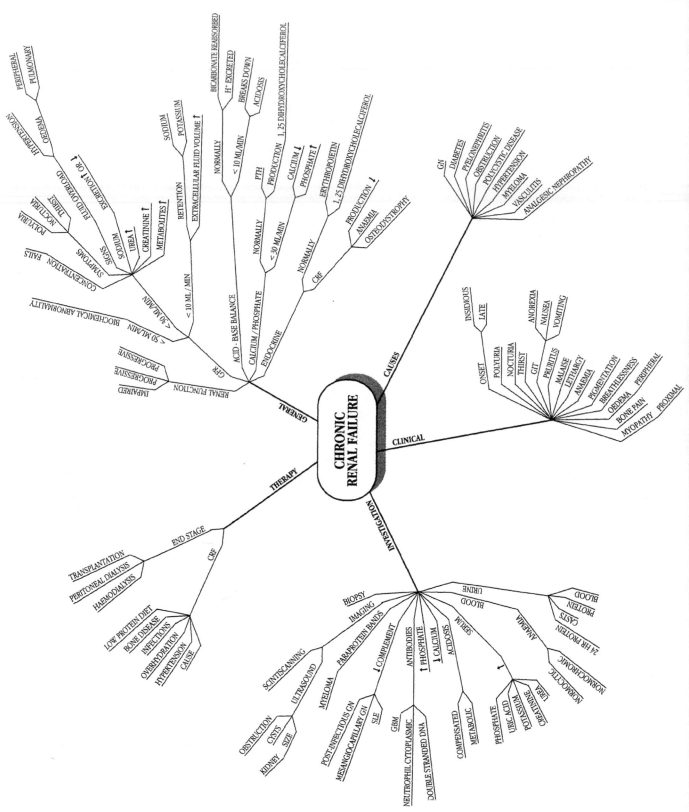

CHRONIC RENAL FAILURE

GLOMERULAR DISEASE

CLINICAL

PATHOLOGY

- IMMUNE INJURY
- SYNDROMES
  - NEPHROTIC SY
    - PROTEINURIA
    - OEDEMA
    - HYPO...
    - PERSISTENT PROTEINURIA
    - <2.0 G/DAY
    - HAEMATURIA
    - FEW --> CRF
  - ACUTE GN
    - FOLLOWS
    - GRADUAL
    - OEDEMA
    - HYPERTENSION
    - RENAL FAILURE
  - CHRONIC GN
  - EXCRETION ↑
    - SALT
    - WATER
    - CAUSING
  - GFR ↓
    - PROTEINURIA
    - HAEMATURIA
    - RED CELL CASTS

INVESTIGATION

GENERAL
- IMMUNE MEDIATED
- CRF COMMONEST CAUSE
- THERAPY SYMPTOMATIC

GENERAL FEATURES

SECONDARY GN
- SBE
- GOODPASTURE'S SY
- HENOCH-SCHONLEIN PURPURA
- PN
- SLE

PRIMARY ACUTE GN

GENERAL
- MOST COMMON GN — GROUP A
- STREPTOCOCCUS — B HAEMOLYTIC
- CHILDREN
- LATENT PERIOD — 10-20 DAYS

INVESTIGATION
- BIOPSY
  - PROLIFERATION
    - MESANGIUM
    - ENDOTHELIUM
  - POLYMORPHS IN GLOMERULI
  - DEPOSITS
    - GBM
    - IgG
    - C3
- ANTIBODY TITRES
  - ASO
  - RISING

PROGNOSIS
- MOST RESOLUTION
- FEW CRF

THERAPY
- LOW SALT DIET
- PROTEIN RESTRICTION
- ANTIHYPERTENSIVES
- ANTIBIOTICS
- DIURETICS
- DIALYSIS

IMMUNE INJURY
- ANTI GBM AB
- IMMUNE COMPLEX DEPOSITION
- POST STREPTOCOCCAL GN
- IN SITU IMMUNE COMPLEX FORMATION
  - SLE
  - GOODPASTURE'S SY
- MEMBRANOUS GLOMERULONEPHROPATHY
- MESANGIUM
- BASEMENT MEMBRANE

ENVIRONMENTAL FACTORS
- INFECTIONS
  - STREPTOCOCCI
  - STAPHYLOCOCCI
  - HEPATITIS B
- TOXINS/DRUGS
  - GOODPASTURE'S SY
    - GLUE
    - PETROL
    - HYDROCARBONS
  - MEMBRANOUS GN
    - CAPTOPRIL
    - PENICILLAMINE
    - GOLD
  - POST STREPTOCOCCAL GN
- SOCIAL DEPRIVATION

GENETIC FACTORS
- HLA
- COMPLEMENT DEFICIENCIES
  - GOODPASTURE'S GN
  - MEMBRANOUS GN
  - C2
  - C4
  - 50% --> GN
- FAMILIAL — MINIMAL CHANGE

INVESTIGATION (BIOPSY)
- STIX TEST
  - PROTEIN
  - BLOOD
- URINE
  - 24 HR PROTEIN
  - CREATININE — PLASMA
- GFR MEASUREMENT
- ANTIBODIES
  - ANTI DOUBLE STRANDED DNA
  - GLOMERULAR BASEMENT MEMBRANE
  - ANTI NEUTROPHIL
- C3 & 4
- LEVELS
  - Ig
    - G
    - A
    - M
- BIOPSY
  - KIDNEY
  - LIGHT MICROSCOPY
  - IMMUNOFLUORESCENCE
  - ELECTRON MICROSCOPY
  - COMPLICATIONS
    - HAEMORRHAGE
    - 1%
  - CONTRAINDICATIONS
    - SINGLE KIDNEY
    - BLEEDING DIATHESIS

MINIMAL CHANGE GN

GENERAL
- NEPHROTIC SY
  - COMMONEST CAUSE
  - 80% CHILDREN
  - 20% ADULTS
- M > F
- PROTEINURIA — MASSIVE > 3 G

ASSOCIATION
- INFECTION
- ALLERGY
- SYSTEMIC DISEASE
  - SLE
  - PN
  - SARCOIDOSIS
  - AMYLOIDOSIS
  - DIABETES MELLITUS
- DRUGS
  - D - PENICILLAMINE
  - CAPTOPRIL
  - HEAVY METALS
- TUMOURS — NOT IN CHILDREN

INVESTIGATION
- BIOPSY
  - LIGHT MICROSCOPY — NORMAL
  - EM
    - FOOT PROCESS FUSION
    - COMPLEX DEPOSITION

THERAPY
- STEROIDS
- CYCLOPHOSPHAMIDE
- CHLORAMBUCIL

PROGNOSIS
- GOOD
- 50% RELAPSE

FOCAL GLOMERULOSCLEROSIS

GENERAL
- NEPHROTIC SY
  - 10% CHILDREN
  - 15% ADULTS

INVESTIGATION
- BIOPSY
  - GLOMERULI
    - SEGMENTAL SCLEROSIS
    - MESANGIAL MATRIX ↑
    - HYALINOSIS
  - COMPLICATIONS
    - IMMUNOGLOBULIN
    - COMPLEMENT
- COURSE
  - 50% IDIOPATHIC
  - 30% ADULTS
  - RARE CHILDREN
  - NEPHROTIC SY
  - IN 75% OF MEMBRANOUS GN

THERAPY
- DIURETICS
- ANTIHYPERTENSIVES
- IMMUNOSUPPRESSIVES

MEMBRANOUS GN

GENERAL
- AS MEMBRANOUS GN
- 10 % OF NEPHROTIC SY
- < 30 YRS

ASSOCIATIONS
- INFECTIONS
  - HEPATITIS B
  - MALARIA
  - BOWEL
  - BRONCHUS
- MALIGNANCY
- DRUGS
  - MERCURY
  - PENICILLAMINE
  - GOLD
- CTD
  - SLE
  - MCTD
  - CRF
- PERSISTENT PROTEINURIA
  - 1.5 YRS
  - 50% REMISSION
  - 25%
  - 25%

INVESTIGATION
- BIOPSY
  - IN SITU COMPLEX FORMATION
  - DEPOSITS
    - IgG
    - C3

THERAPY
- IMMUNOSUPRESSION
- STEROIDS
- CAUSE

MESANGIOCAPILLARY GN

GENERAL
- 10 - 50YRS
- MALES
- URTI
- RECURRENT

ASSOCIATIONS
- INFECTIONS

INVESTIGATION
- BIOPSY
  - DEPOSITS
    - TYPE 1
    - TYPE 2
      - IN GBM
      - NOT Ig
      - DENSE
  - CAPILLARY WALL — THICKENED
  - MESANGIUM PROLIFERATION
    - MATRIX
    - CELLS
- SERUM
  - C3 NEPHRITIC FACTOR
    - C3 ↓
    - HYPOCOMPLEMENTAEMIA
    - AUTOANTIBODY
    - C3 CONVERTASE INHIBITOR
    - IgG

THERAPY
- SYMPTOMATIC

IGA NEPHROPATHY

GENERAL
- 10 - 50YRS
- MALES
- RECURRENT
- URTI

ASSOCIATIONS
- INFECTIONS

INVESTIGATION
- BIOPSY
  - DEPOSITS
    - IgA
    - MESANGIUM
  - SCLEROSIS
    - FOCAL
    - SEGMENTAL

THERAPY
- SYMPTOMATIC
- TRANSPLANT — MAY RECUR IN

PROGNOSIS
- CRF 15%

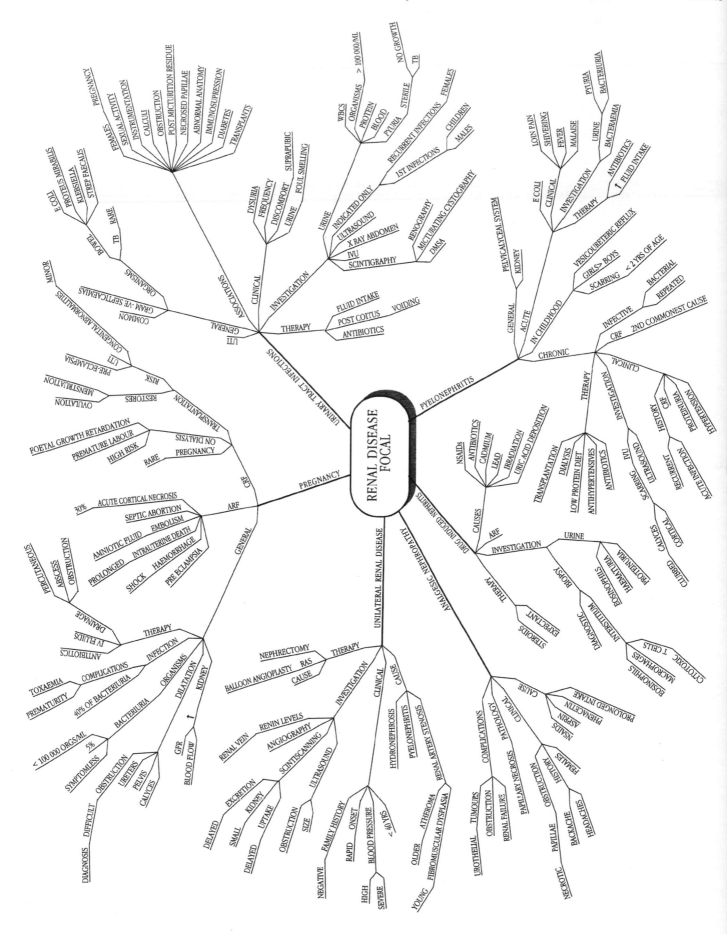

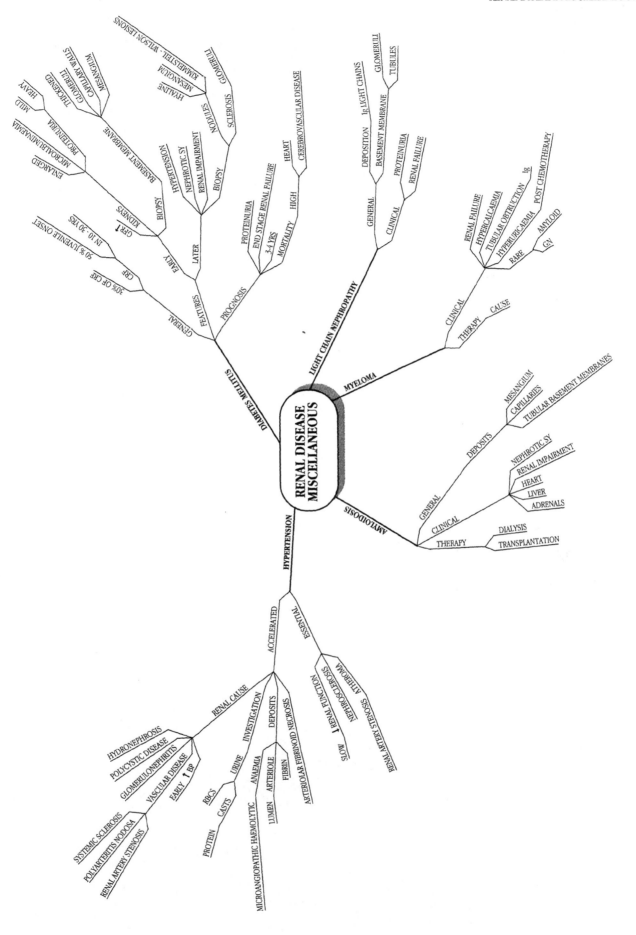

RENAL DISEASE MISCELLANEOUS

DIABETES MELLITUS
- GENERAL
  - FEATURES
    - PROTEINURIA
      - MICROALBUMINAEMIA
        - MILD
      - PROTEINURIA
        - HEAVY
    - BASEMENT MEMBRANE
      - GLOMERULI THICKENED
      - CAPILLARY WALLS
    - MESANGIUM
      - HYALINE
      - KIMMELSTIEL - WILSON LESIONS
    - GLOMERULI
      - NODULES
      - SCLEROSIS
    - ENLARGED KIDNEYS
      - CRF ↑ EARLY
      - CRF ↓ LATER
        - 30% OF CRF
        - IN 10 - 30 YRS
        - 50 % JUVENILE ONSET
    - BIOPSY
      - HYPERTENSION
      - NEPHROTIC SY
      - RENAL IMPAIRMENT
      - BIOPSY
  - PROGNOSIS
    - END STAGE RENAL FAILURE
      - 3-4 YRS
    - MORTALITY
      - HIGH
      - HEART
      - CEREBROVASCULAR DISEASE

LIGHT CHAIN NEPHROPATHY
- GENERAL
  - DEPOSITION Ig LIGHT CHAINS
    - BASEMENT MEMBRANE
      - GLOMERULI
      - TUBULES
- CLINICAL
  - PROTEINURIA
  - RENAL FAILURE

MYELOMA
- CLINICAL
  - RENAL FAILURE
    - HYPERCALCAEMIA
      - TUBULAR OBSTRUCTION
    - HYPERURICAEMIA
      - POST CHEMOTHERAPY
      - Ig
    - RARE
      - AMYLOID
      - GN
- THERAPY
- CAUSE

AMYLOIDOSIS
- GENERAL
  - DEPOSITS
    - MESANGIUM
    - CAPILLARIES
    - TUBULAR BASEMENT MEMBRANES
- CLINICAL
  - NEPHROTIC SY
  - RENAL IMPAIRMENT
  - HEART
  - LIVER
  - ADRENALS
- THERAPY
  - DIALYSIS
  - TRANSPLANTATION

HYPERTENSION
- ACCELERATED
  - RENAL CAUSE
    - HYDRONEPHROSIS
    - POLYCYSTIC DISEASE
    - GLOMERULONEPHRITIS
    - VASCULAR DISEASE
      - SYSTEMIC SCLEROSIS
      - POLYARTERITIS NODOSA
      - RENAL ARTERY STENOSIS
    - EARLY ↑ BP
  - INVESTIGATION
    - URINE
      - RBCS
      - CASTS
      - PROTEIN
    - ANAEMIA
      - MICROANGIOPATHIC HAEMOLYTIC
    - DEPOSITS
      - ARTERIOLE
        - LUMEN
        - FIBRIN
      - ARTERIOLAR FIBRINOID NECROSIS
- ESSENTIAL
  - NEPHROSCLEROSIS
    - ATHEROMA
    - ↑ RENAL FUNCTION
      - SLOW
    - RENAL ARTERY STENOSIS

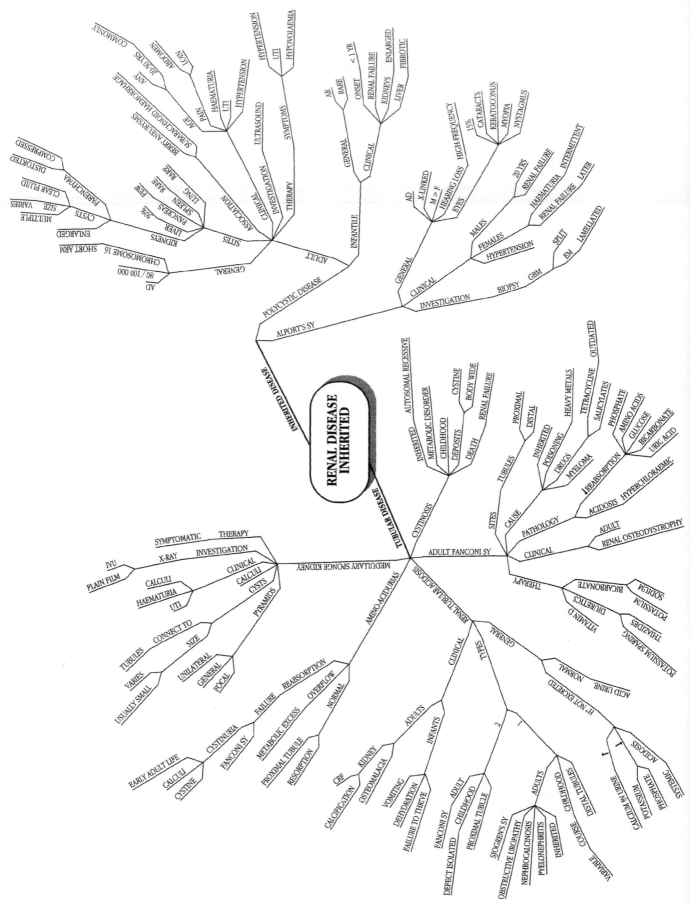

RENAL DISEASE INHERITED

Nutrition

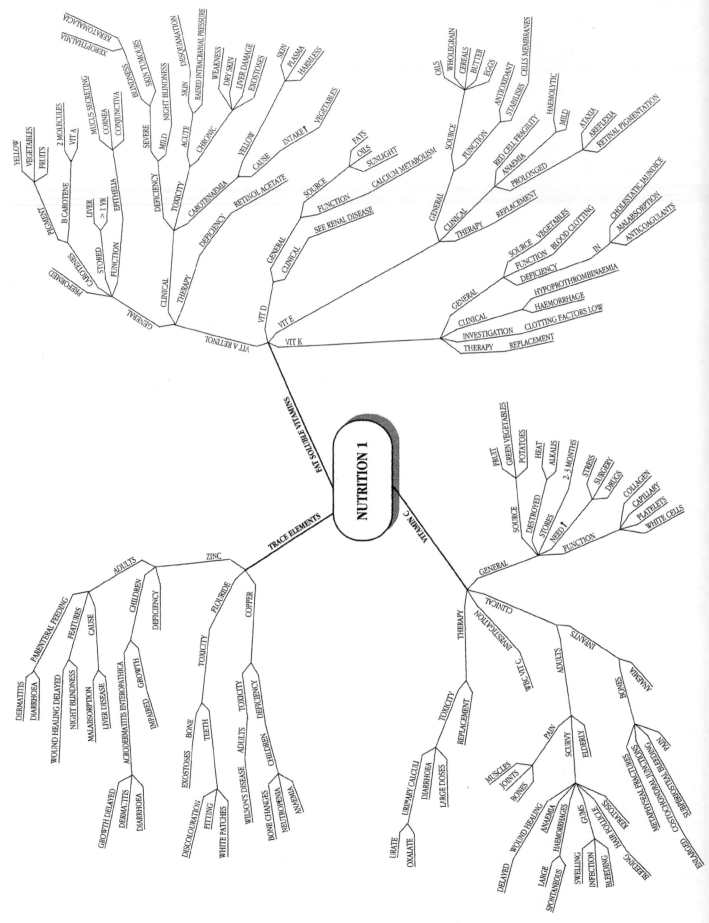

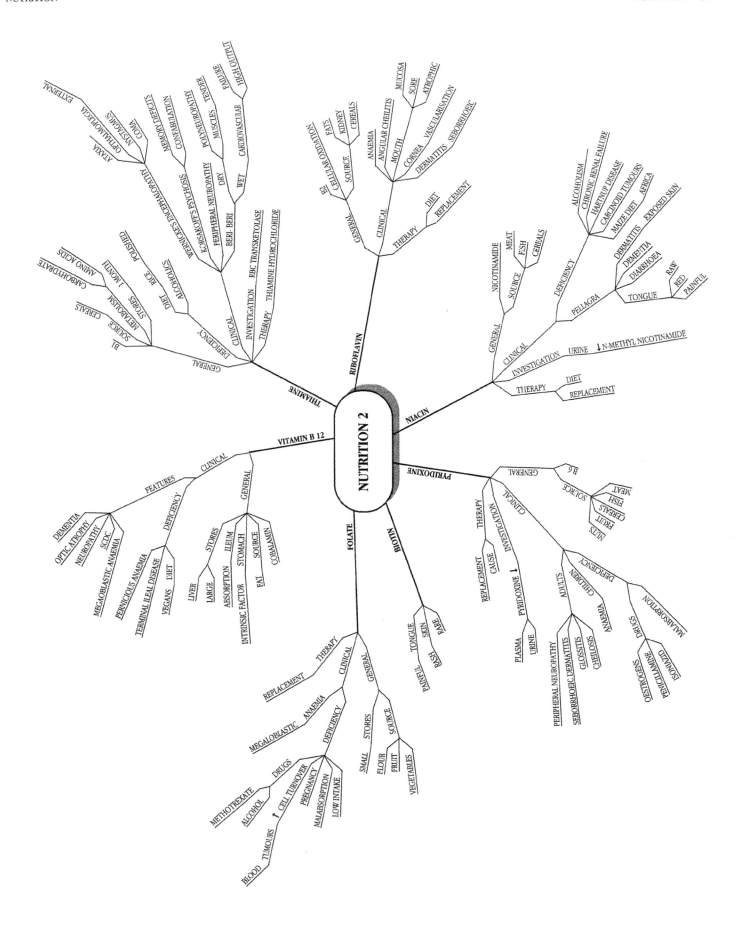

Gastrointestinal tract

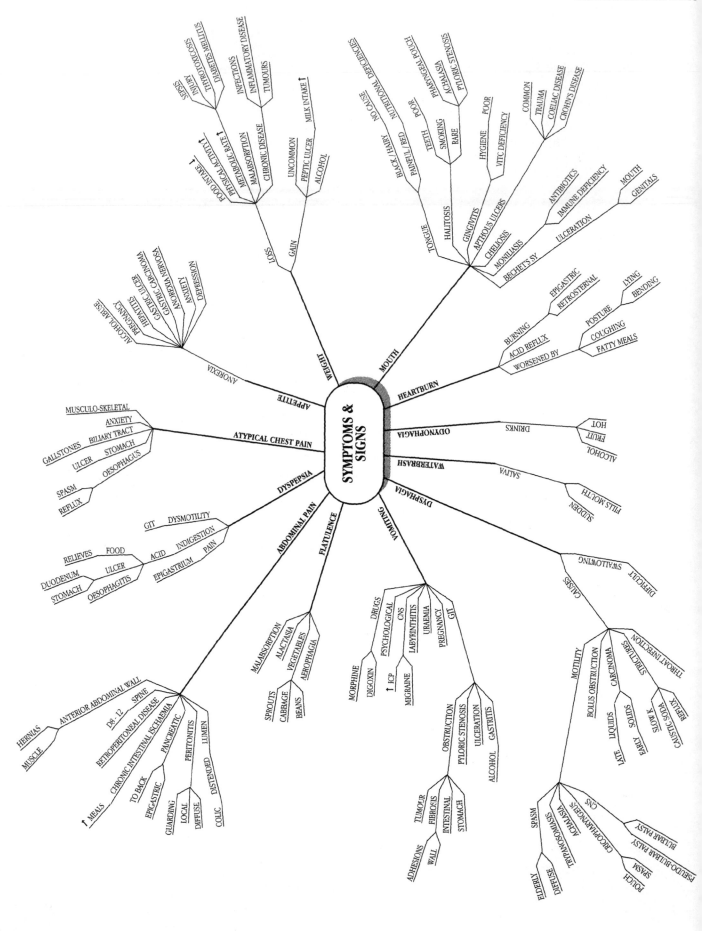

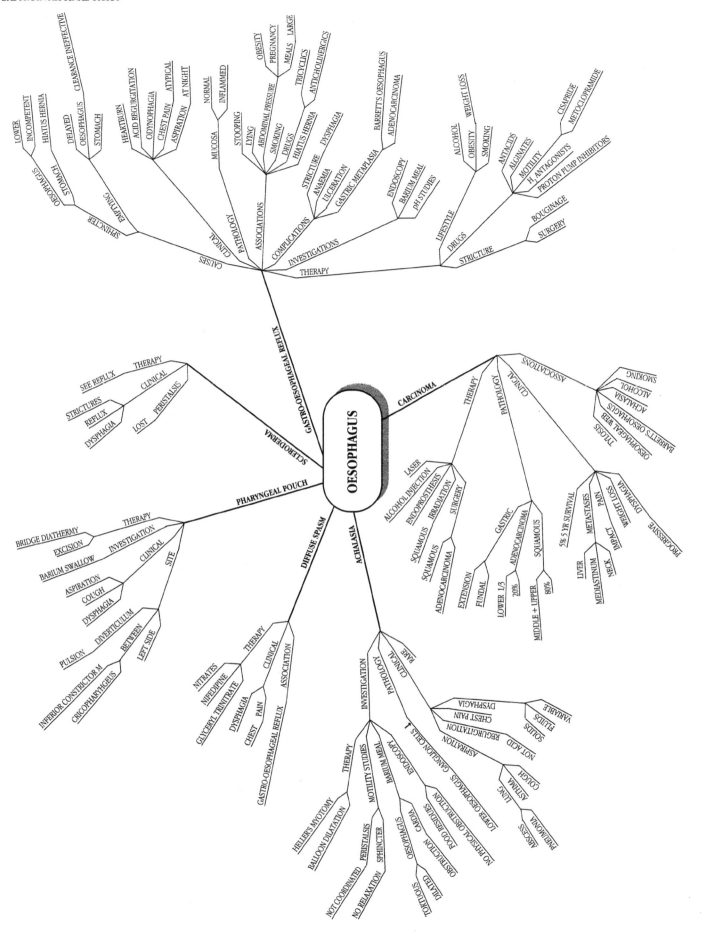

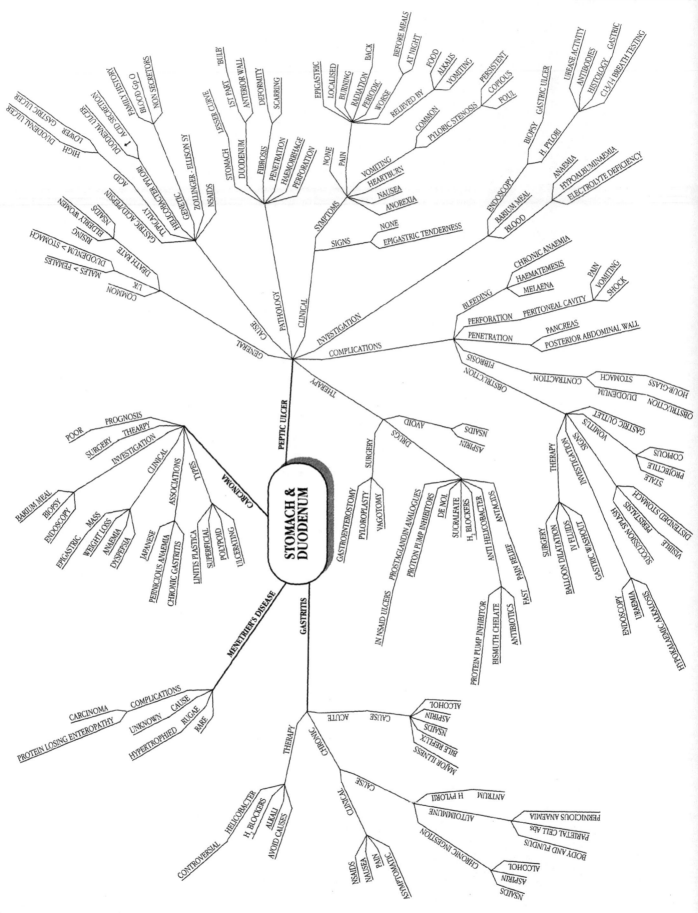

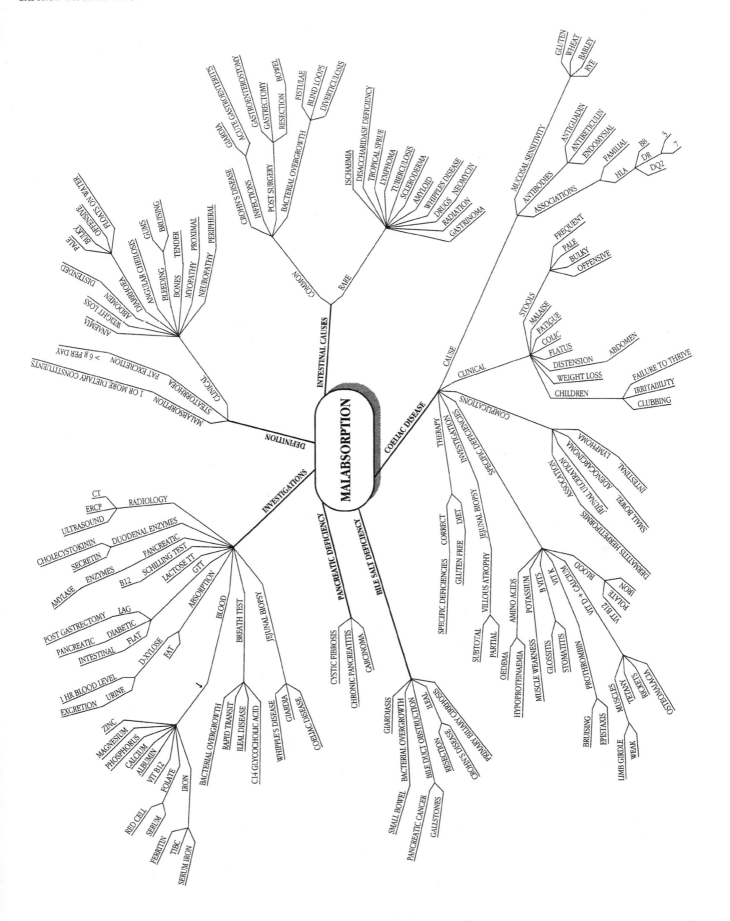

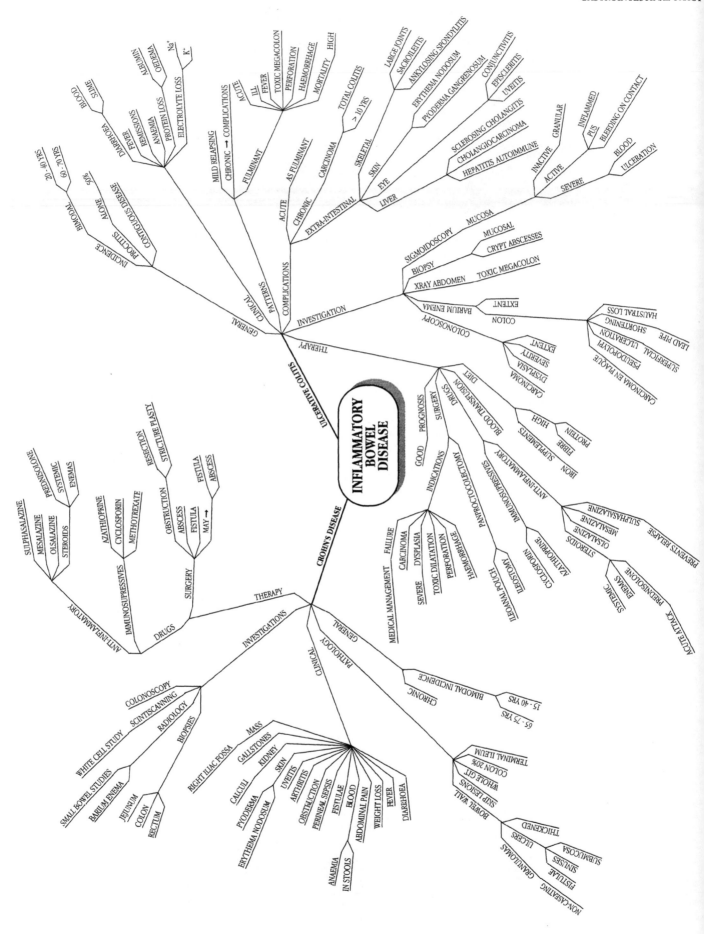

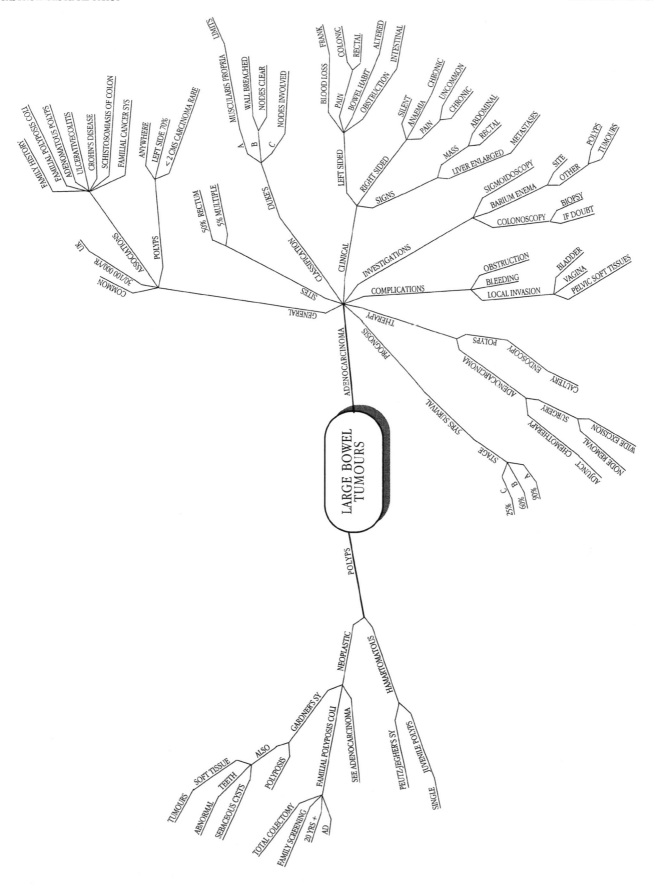

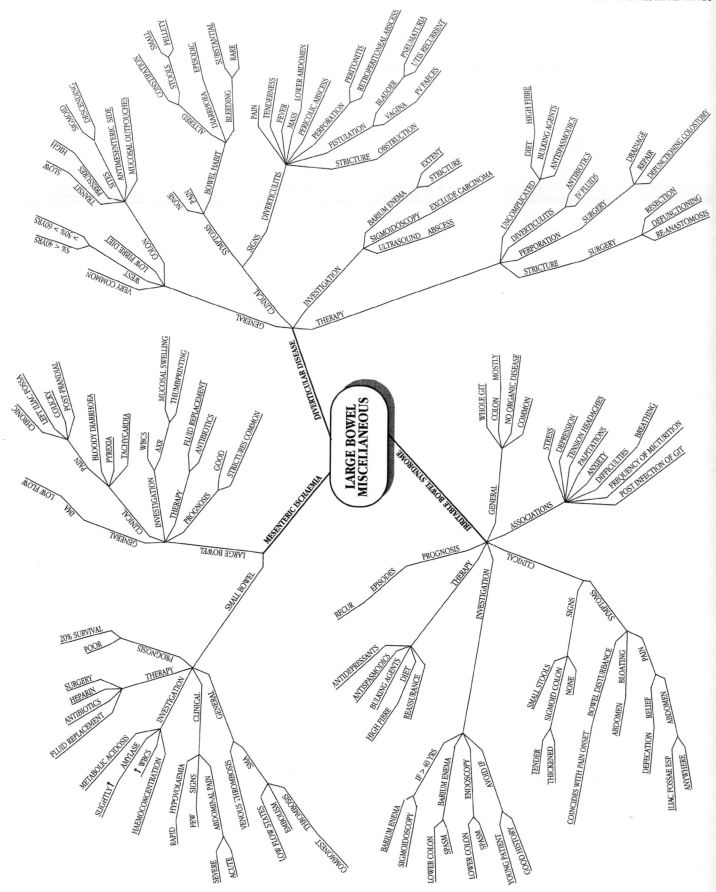

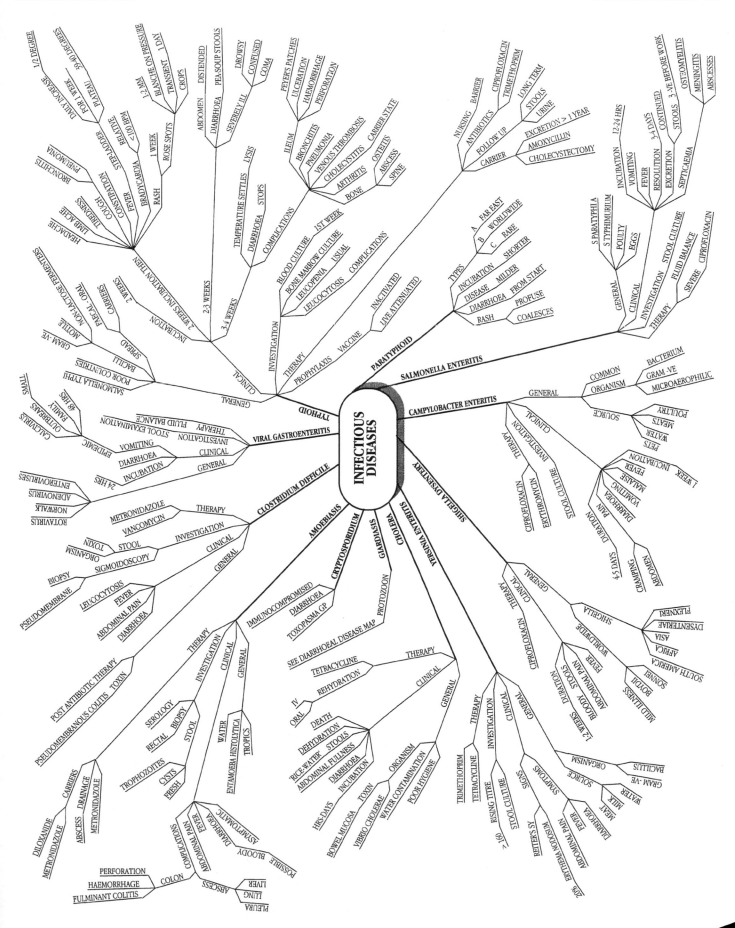

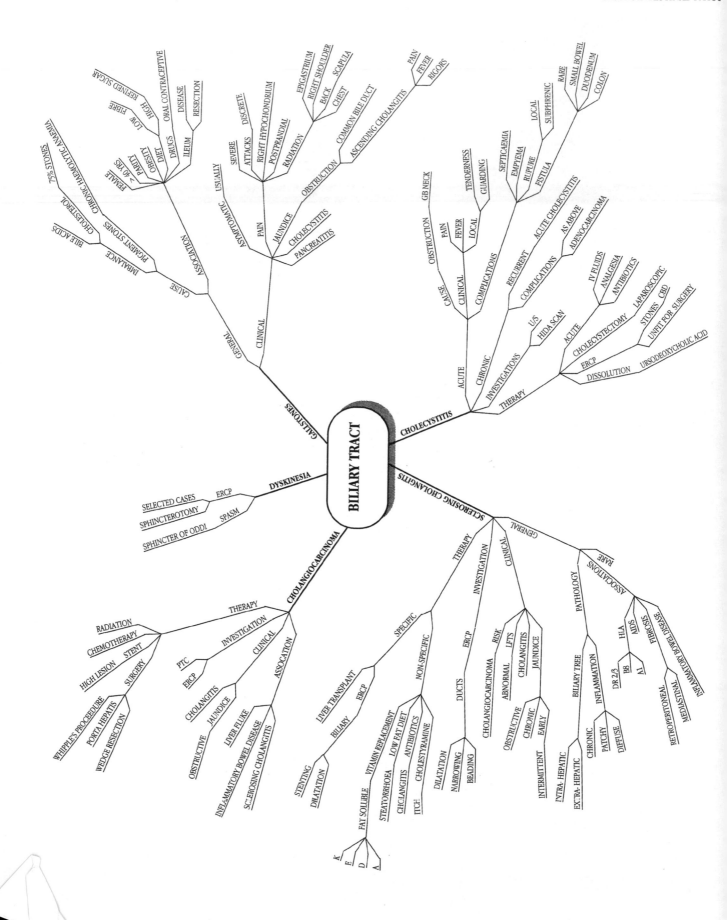

BILIARY TRACT

GALLSTONES

CAUSE
- ASSOCIATION
  - FEMALE
  - > 40 YRS
  - PARITY
  - OBESITY
  - DIET
    - HIGH REFINED SUGAR
    - LOW FIBRE
    - HIGH
  - DRUGS
    - ORAL CONTRACEPTIVE
  - DISEASE
    - ILEUM
    - RESECTION
- IMBALANCE
  - PIGMENT STONES
    - 25% STONES
    - CHRONIC HAEMOLYTIC ANAEMIA
  - CHOLESTEROL
    - 75% STONES
  - BILE ACIDS

CLINICAL
- GENERAL
  - ASYMPTOMATIC
    - USUALLY
  - PAIN
    - JAUNDICE
    - CHOLECYSTITIS
    - PANCREATITIS
- PAIN
  - SEVERE
  - DISCRETE
  - ATTACKS
  - RIGHT HYPOCHONDRIUM
  - POSTPRANDIAL
  - EPIGASTRIUM
  - RIGHT SHOULDER
  - BACK
  - SCAPULA
  - CHEST
- JAUNDICE
  - OBSTRUCTION
    - RADIATION
    - COMMON BILE DUCT
  - ASCENDING CHOLANGITIS
    - PAIN
    - FEVER
    - RIGORS

CHOLECYSTITIS
- ACUTE
  - CAUSE
    - OBSTRUCTION
      - GB NECK
  - CLINICAL
    - PAIN
    - FEVER
      - LOCAL
    - TENDERNESS
    - GUARDING
  - COMPLICATIONS
    - SEPTICAEMIA
    - EMPYEMA
    - RUPURE
    - FISTULA
      - LOCAL
      - SUBPHRENIC
      - RARE
      - SMALL BOWEL
      - DUODENUM
      - COLON
- CHRONIC
  - RECURRENT
  - ACUTE CHOLECYSTITIS
  - COMPLICATIONS
    - AS ABOVE
    - ADENOCARCINOMA
- INVESTIGATIONS
  - U/S
  - HIDA SCAN
- THERAPY
  - ACUTE
    - IV FLUIDS
    - ANALGESIA
    - ANTIBIOTICS
  - CHOLECYSTECTOMY
    - LAPAROSCOPIC
    - ERCP
      - STONES
      - CBD
      - UNFIT FOR SURGERY
  - DISSOLUTION
    - URSODEOXYCHOLIC ACID

DYSKINESIA
- ERCP
  - SELECTED CASES
- SPASM
  - SPHINCTEROTOMY
  - SPHINCTER OF ODDI

CHOLANGIOCARCINOMA
- THERAPY
  - RADIATION
  - CHEMOTHERAPY
  - STENT
    - HIGH LESION
  - SURGERY
    - WHIPPLES PROCEDURE
    - PORTA HEPATIS
    - WEDGE RESECTION
- INVESTIGATION
  - PTC
  - ERCP
- CLINICAL
  - CHOLANGITIS
  - JAUNDICE
    - OBSTRUCTIVE
- ASSOCIATION
  - LIVER FLUKE
  - INFLAMMATORY BOWEL DISEASE
  - SCLEROSING CHOLANGITIS

SCLEROSING CHOLANGITIS
- THERAPY
  - LIVER TRANSPLANT
  - STENTING
  - DILATATION
  - SPECIFIC
    - BILIARY
  - NON-SPECIFIC
    - VITAMIN REPLACEMENT
      - FAT SOLUBLE
        - K
        - E
        - D
        - A
    - LOW FAT DIET
      - STEATORRHOEA
    - ANTIBIOTICS
      - CHOLANGITIS
    - CHOLESTYRAMINE
      - ITCH
- INVESTIGATION
  - ERCP
    - DUCTS
      - DILATATION
      - NARROWING
      - BEADING
- CLINICAL
  - RISK
    - CHOLANGIOCARCINOMA
  - LFTS
    - ABNORMAL
  - CHOLANGITIS
  - JAUNDICE
    - OBSTRUCTIVE
    - CHRONIC
    - INTERMITTENT
    - EARLY
- GENERAL
  - PATHOLOGY
    - BILIARY TREE
      - INTRA- HEPATIC
      - EXTRA- HEPATIC
    - INFLAMMATION
      - CHRONIC
      - PATCHY
      - DIFFUSE
  - ASSOCIATIONS
    - HLA
      - DR 2/3
      - B8
      - A1
    - AIDS
    - FIBROSIS
      - RETROPERITONEAL
      - MEDIASTINAL
    - INFLAMMATORY BOWEL DISEASE
  - RARE

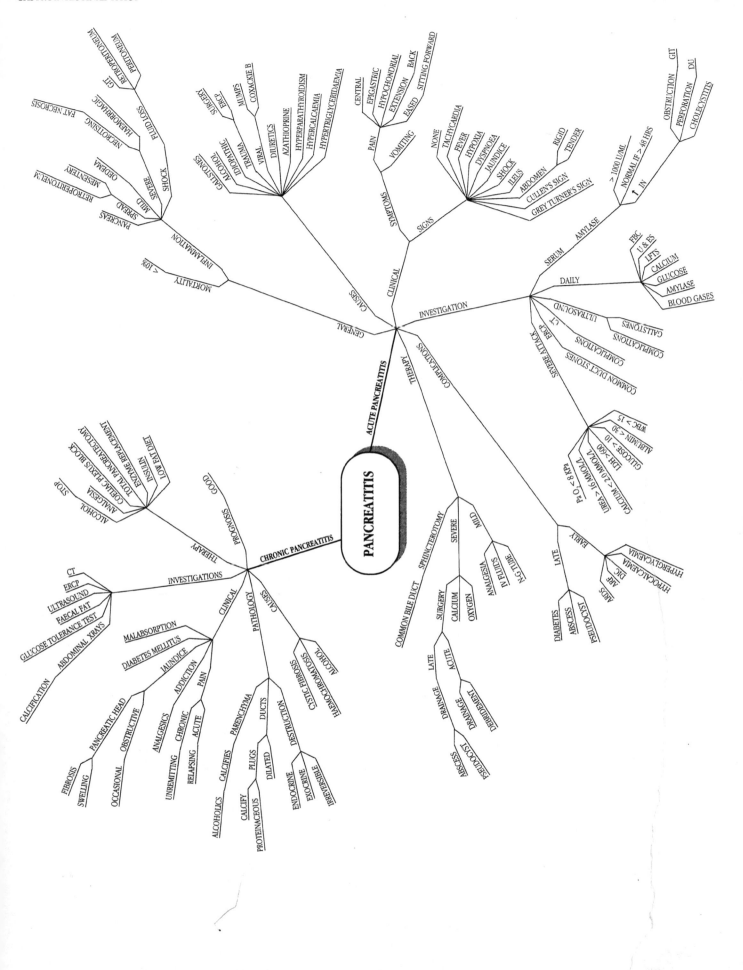

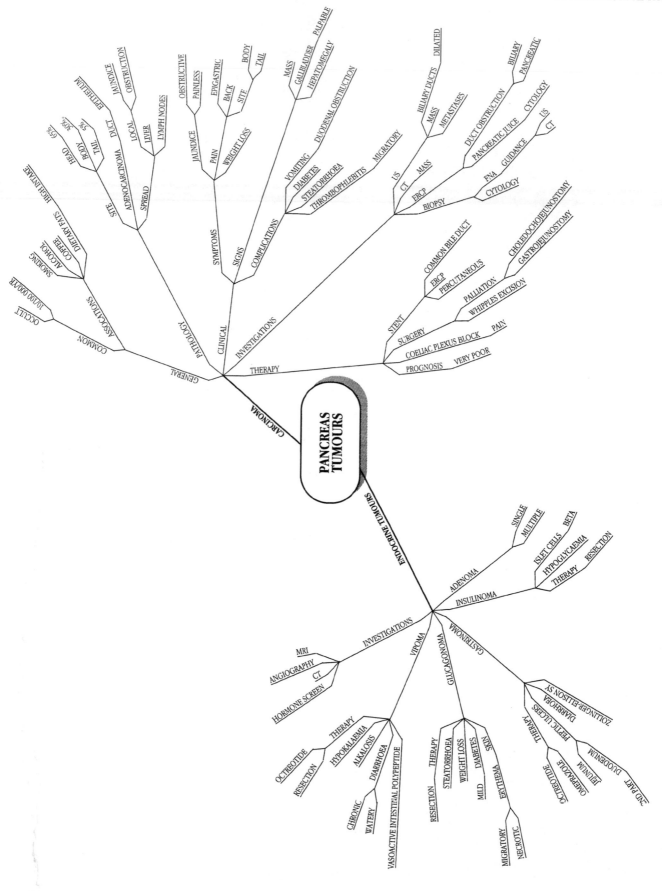

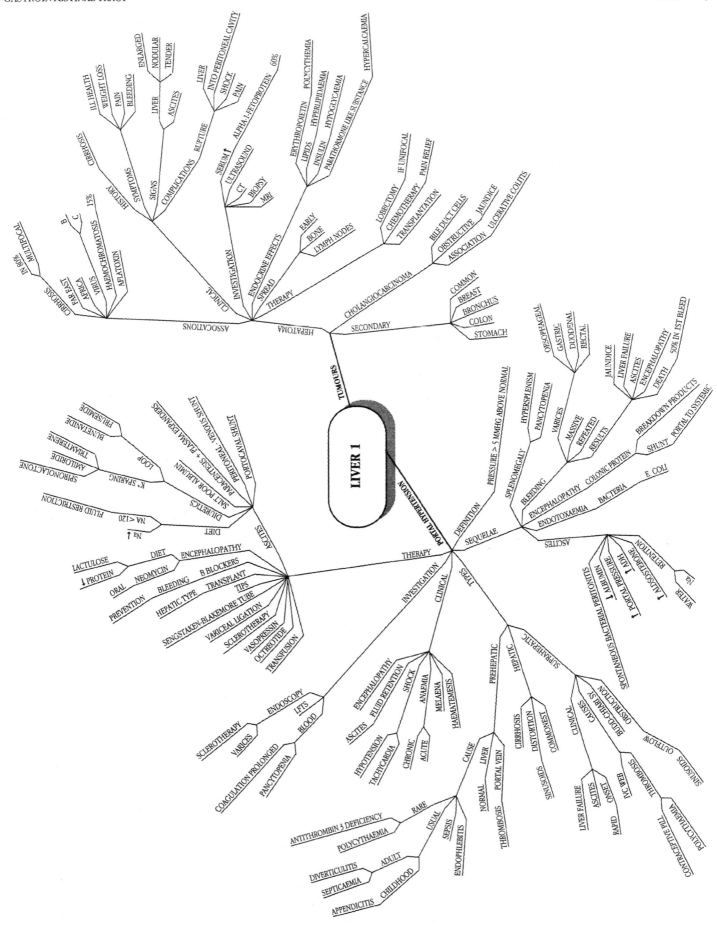

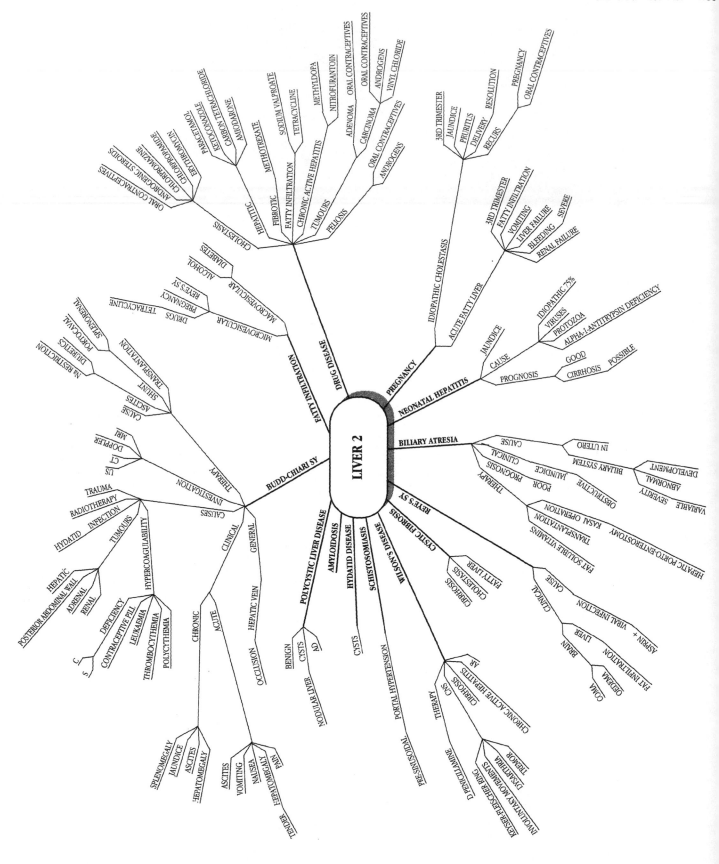

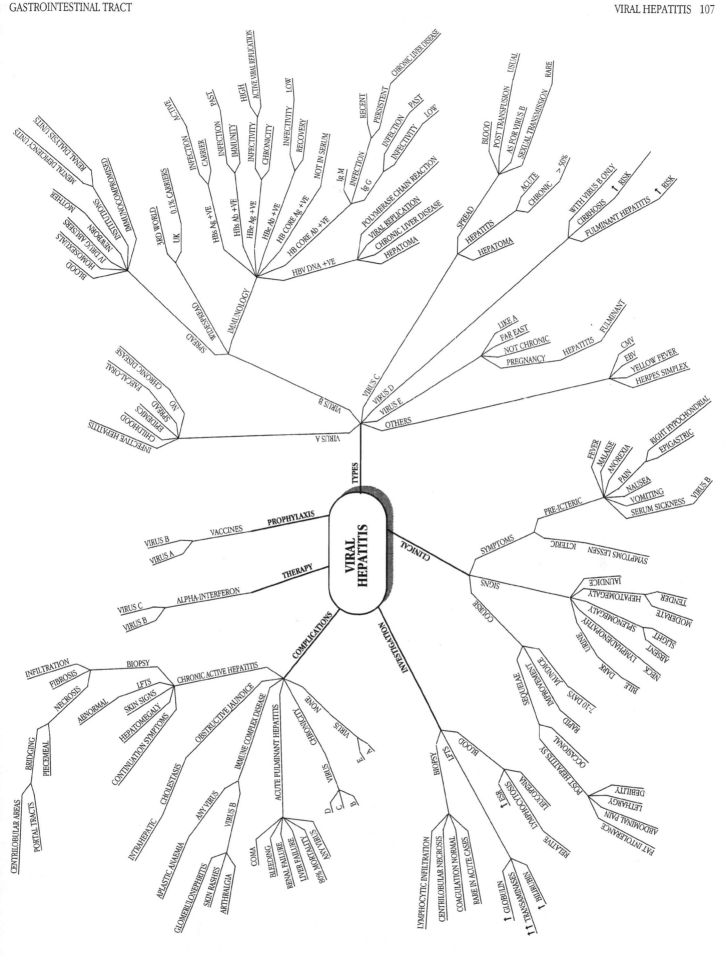

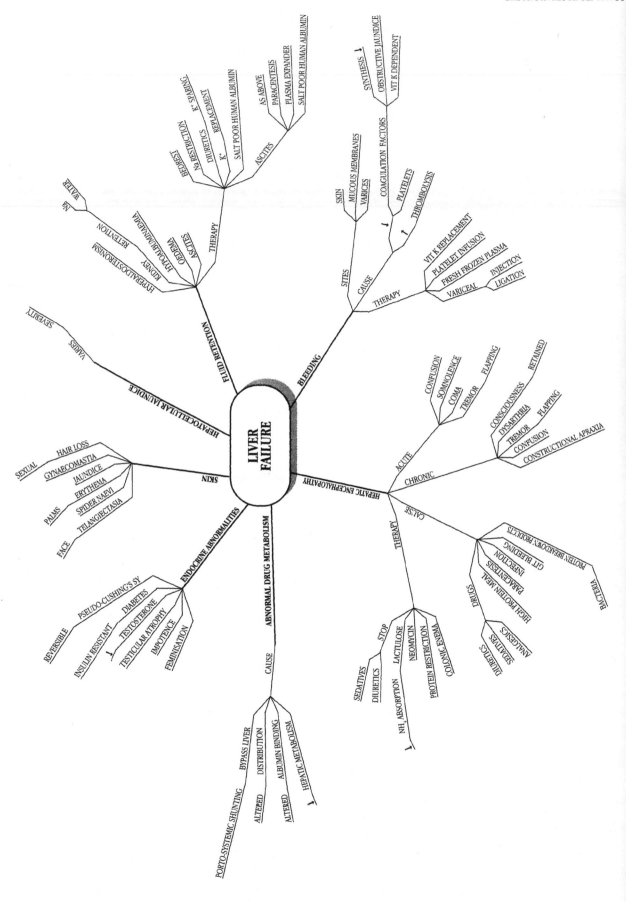

LIVER FAILURE

FLUID RETENTION

THERAPY
ASCITES — BEDREST — Na RESTRICTION — DIURETICS — K⁺ — K⁺ SPARING — SALT POOR HUMAN ALBUMIN — REPLACEMENT — AS ABOVE — PARACENTESIS — PLASMA EXPANDER — SALT POOR HUMAN ALBUMIN

ASCITES — OEDEMA — HYPOALBUMINAEMIA — KIDNEY — HYPERALDOSTERONISM — RETENTION — Na — WATER

HEPATOCELLULAR JAUNDICE
VARIES — SEVERITY

BLEEDING
SITES — SKIN — MUCOUS MEMBRANES — VARICES
CAUSE — COAGULATION FACTORS — SYNTHESIS — OBSTRUCTIVE JAUNDICE — VIT K DEPENDENT — PLATELETS — THROMBOLYSIS
THERAPY — VIT K REPLACEMENT — PLATELET INFUSION — FRESH FROZEN PLASMA — VARICEAL — INJECTION — LIGATION

HEPATIC ENCEPHALOPATHY
ACUTE — CONFUSION — SOMNOLENCE — COMA — TREMOR — FLAPPING
CHRONIC — CONSCIOUSNESS — RETAINED — DYSARTHRIA — FLAPPING — TREMOR — CONFUSION — CONSTRUCTIONAL APRAXIA
CAUSE — PROTEIN BREAKDOWN PRODUCTS — GIT BLEEDING — INFECTION — PARACENTESIS — HIGH PROTEIN MEAL — DRUGS — DIURETICS — SEDATIVES — ANALGESICS — BACTERIA
THERAPY — SEDATIVES — DIURETICS — STOP — LACTULOSE — NEOMYCIN — COLONIC ENEMA — PROTEIN RESTRICTION — NH₃ ABSORPTION

ABNORMAL DRUG METABOLISM
CAUSE — PORTO-SYSTEMIC SHUNTING — BYPASS LIVER — DISTRIBUTION — ALTERED — ALBUMIN BINDING — HEPATIC METABOLISM — ALTERED

ENDOCRINE ABNORMALITIES
PSEUDO-CUSHING'S SY — REVERSIBLE — DIABETES — INSULIN RESISTANT — TESTOSTERONE — TESTICULAR ATROPHY — IMPOTENCE — FEMINISATION

SKIN
SEXUAL — HAIR LOSS — GYNAECOMASTIA — JAUNDICE — ERYTHEMA — PALMS — SPIDER NAEVI — FACE — TELANGIECTASIA

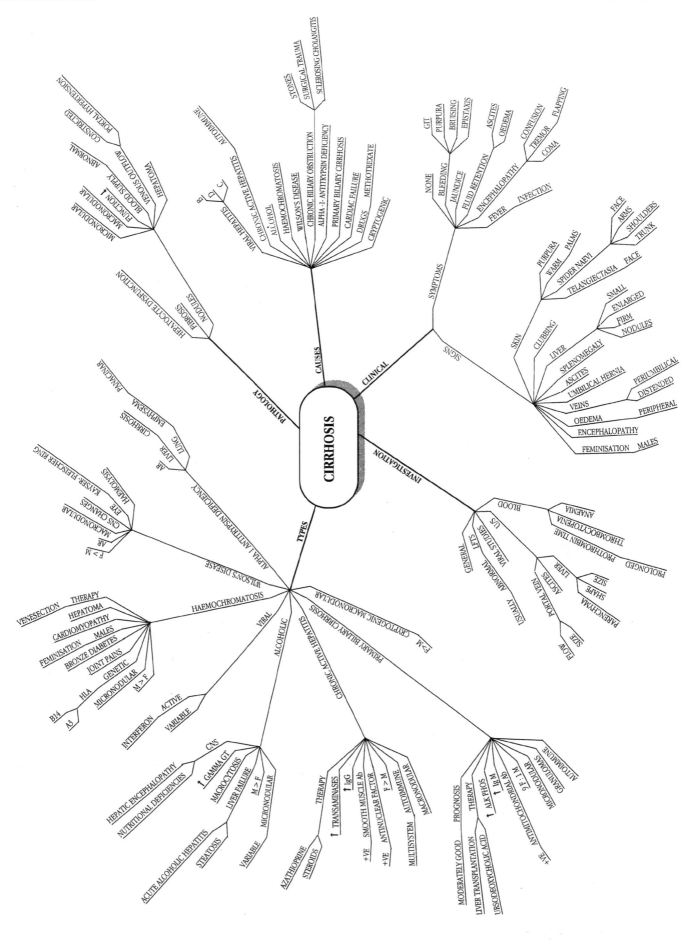

CIRRHOSIS

PATHOLOGY

CAUSES

Fibrosis

Nodules

Hepatocyte dysfunction

Hepatoma

Macronodular

Micronodular

Portal hypertension

Constricted

Abnormal

Blood supply

Venous outflow

Function ↑

Viral hepatitis

Chronic active hepatitis

Alcohol

Haemochromatosis

Wilson's disease

Chronic biliary obstruction

Alpha-1-antitrypsin deficiency

Primary biliary cirrhosis

Cardiac failure

Methotrexate

Drugs

Cryptogenic

Autoimmune

A B C

Stones

Surgical trauma

Sclerosing cholangitis

CLINICAL

SYMPTOMS

None

Bleeding

Jaundice

Fluid retention

Encephalopathy

Fever

Infection

GIT

Purpura

Bruising

Epistaxis

Ascites

Oedema

Confusion

Flapping

Tremor

Coma

SIGNS

Skin

Clubbing

Liver

Splenomegaly

Ascites

Umbilical hernia

Veins

Oedema

Encephalopathy

Feminisation Males

Purpura

Warm palms

Spider naevi

Telangiectasia Face

Small

Enlarged

Firm

Nodules

Periumbilical

Distended

Peripheral

Face

Arms

Shoulders

Trunk

INVESTIGATION

Blood

U/S

LFTs

Viral studies

General

Usually abnormal

Ascites

Portal vein

Liver

Size

Shape

Flow

Size

Parenchyma

Prolonged

Prothrombin time

Thrombocytopenia

Anaemia

TYPES

Wilson's disease

Alpha 1 antitrypsin deficiency

Haemochromatosis

Viral

Alcoholic

Chronic active hepatitis

Primary biliary cirrhosis

Cryptogenic Macronodular

F > M

Lung

Liver

Emphysema

Cirrhosis

AR

Parencar

AR

Macronodular

CNS changes

Eye

Haemolysis

Kayser Fleischer ring

F > M

Therapy

Venesection

Hepatoma

Cardiomyopathy

Feminisation Males

Bronze diabetes

Joint pains

Genetic

HLA Micronodular M > F

B14

A3

Interferon Active

Variable

CNS

↑ Gamma GT

Macrocytosis

Liver failure M > F

Variable Micronodular

Hepatic encephalopathy

Nutritional deficiencies

Acute alcoholic hepatitis

Steatosis

Therapy

↑ IgG

↑ transaminases

Smooth muscle Ab

Antinuclear factor F > M

Autoimmune

Macronodular

Multisystem

+ve

+ve

Azathioprine

Steroids

Prognosis

Therapy

Alk phos ↑

IgM ↑

Anti-mitochondrial Ab

F : 1 M 9

Micronodular

Granulomas

Autoimmune

Moderately good

Liver transplantation

Ursodeoxycholic acid

+ve

+ve anti-mitochondrial

Metabolic disorders

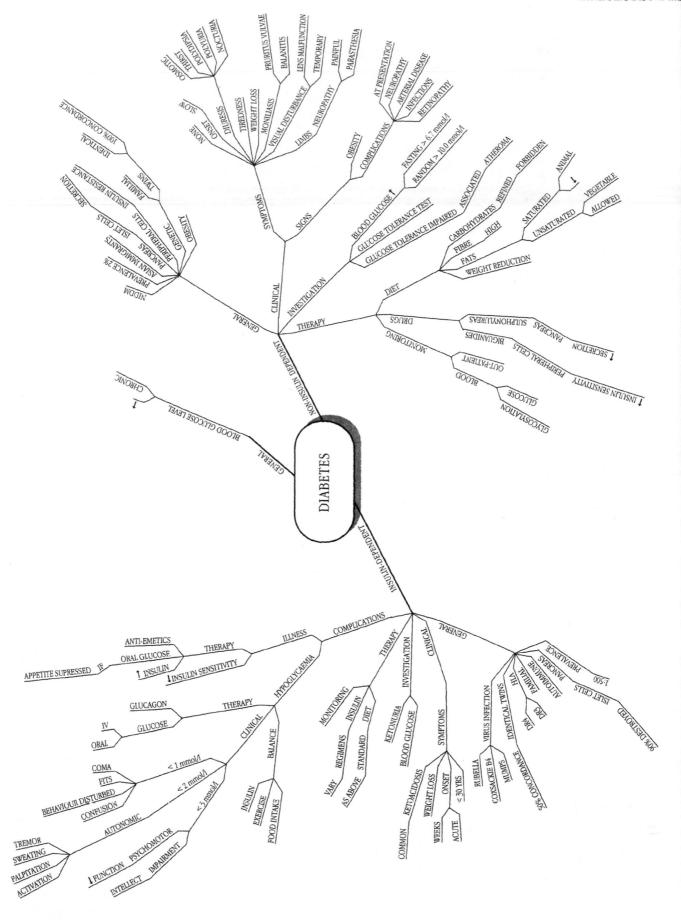

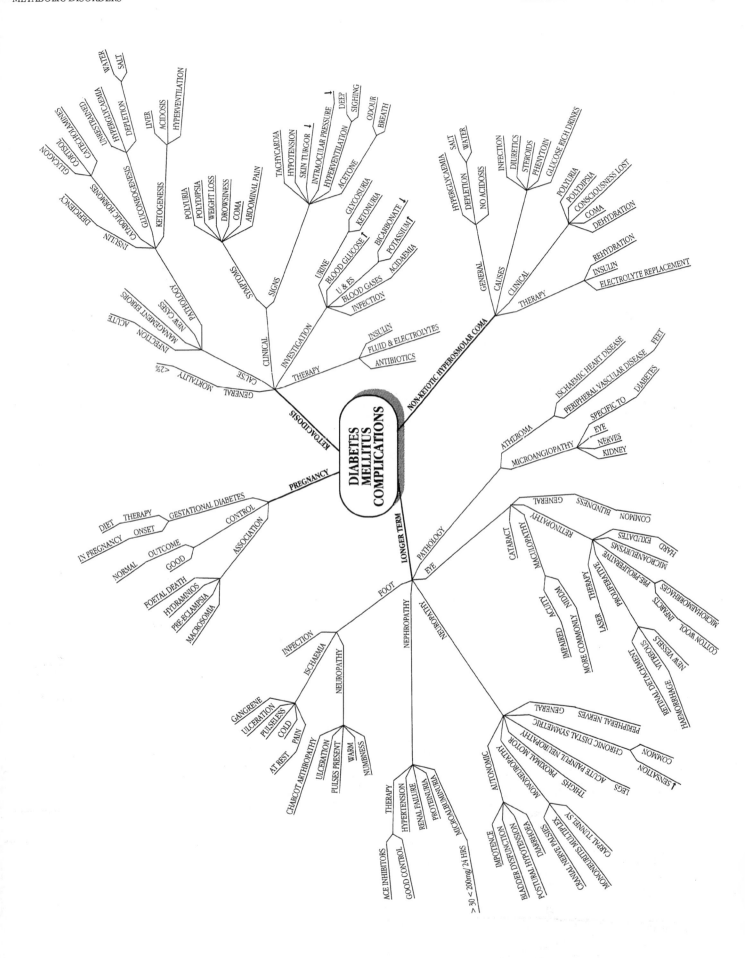

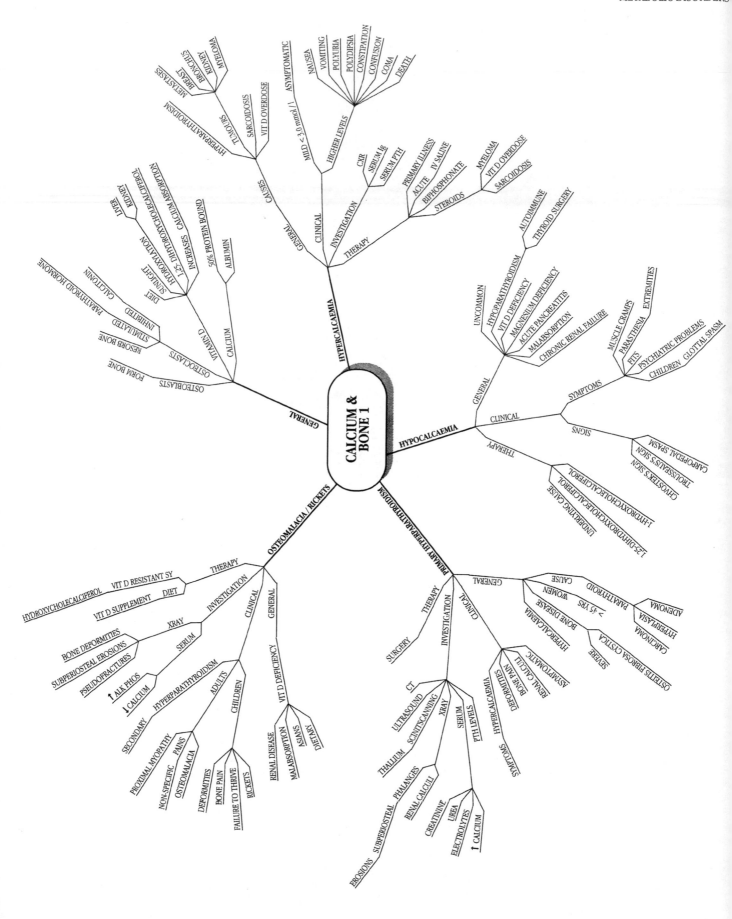

CALCIUM & BONE 1

HYPERCALCAEMIA

GENERAL — CAUSES
- HYPERPARATHYROIDISM
- TUMOURS
  - METASTASES
    - BREAST
    - BRONCHUS
    - KIDNEY
  - MYELOMA
- SARCOIDOSIS
- VIT D OVERDOSE
- MILD < 3.0 mmol /1 — ASYMPTOMATIC

CLINICAL
- HIGHER LEVELS
  - NAUSEA
  - VOMITING
  - POLYURIA
  - POLYDIPSIA
  - CONSTIPATION
  - CONFUSION
  - COMA
  - DEATH

INVESTIGATION
- CXR
- SERUM Ig
- SERUM PTH

THERAPY
- PRIMARY ILLNESS
- IV SALINE
- ACUTE
  - BIPHOSPHONATE
  - STEROIDS
    - MYELOMA
    - VIT D OVERDOSE
    - SARCOIDOSIS

GENERAL

CALCIUM
- INCREASES CALCIUM ABSORPTION — 1.25-DIHYDROXYCHOLECALCIFEROL
  - KIDNEY
  - LIVER
- 50% PROTEIN BOUND — ALBUMIN

VITAMIN D
- 1.25-DIHYDROXYCHOLECALCIFEROL
- 1.25-HYDROXYLATION
- SUNLIGHT
- DIET

OSTEOCLASTS
- CALCITONIN — INHIBITED
- PARATHYROID HORMONE — STIMULATED
- RESORB BONE

OSTEOBLASTS
- FORM BONE

HYPOCALCAEMIA

CLINICAL

GENERAL
- UNCOMMON
- HYPOPARATHYROIDISM
  - AUTOIMMUNE
  - THYROID SURGERY
- VIT D DEFICIENCY
- MAGNESIUM DEFICIENCY
- ACUTE PANCREATITIS
- MALABSORPTION
- CHRONIC RENAL FAILURE

SYMPTOMS
- MUSCLE CRAMPS
- PARASTHESIA — EXTREMITIES
- FITS
- PSYCHIATRIC PROBLEMS
- CHILDREN — GLOTTAL SPASM

SIGNS
- TROUSSEAU'S SIGN — CARPOPEDAL SPASM
- CHVOSTEK'S SIGN

THERAPY
- UNDERLYING CAUSE
- 1-HYDROXYCHOLECALCIFEROL
- 1.25-DIHYDROXYCHOLECALCIFEROL

PRIMARY HYPERPARATHYROIDISM

GENERAL — CAUSE
- PARATHYROID
  - ADENOMA
  - HYPERPLASIA
  - CARCINOMA
- OSTEITIS FIBROSA CYSTICA
- BONE DISEASE
  - SEVERE
  - HYPERCALCAEMIA
- WOMEN — > 45 YRS

CLINICAL
- HYPERCALCAEMIA — SYMPTOMS
- BONE PAIN
- RENAL CALCULI
- DEFORMITIES
- ASYMPTOMATIC

INVESTIGATION
- CT
- ULTRASOUND
- SCINTISCANNING — THALLIUM
- XRAY
  - SUBPERIOSTEAL — PHALANGES
  - EROSIONS
- SERUM
  - RENAL CALCULI
  - CREATININE
  - UREA
  - ELECTROLYTES
  - ↑ CALCIUM
- PTH LEVELS

THERAPY — SURGERY

OSTEOMALACIA / RICKETS

THERAPY
- VIT D RESISTANT SY — HYDROXYCHOLECALCIFEROL
- DIET — VIT D SUPPLEMENT

INVESTIGATION
- XRAY
  - BONE DEFORMITIES
  - SUBPERIOSTEAL EROSIONS
  - PSEUDOFRACTURES
- SERUM
  - ↑ ALK PHOS
  - ↓ CALCIUM
- HYPERPARATHYROIDISM — SECONDARY

CLINICAL
- ADULTS
  - PROXIMAL MYOPATHY
  - PAINS — NON-SPECIFIC
  - OSTEOMALACIA
  - DEFORMITIES
  - BONE PAIN
- CHILDREN
  - RICKETS
  - FAILURE TO THRIVE

GENERAL — VIT D DEFICIENCY
- RENAL DISEASE
- MALABSORPTION
- ASIANS
- DIETARY

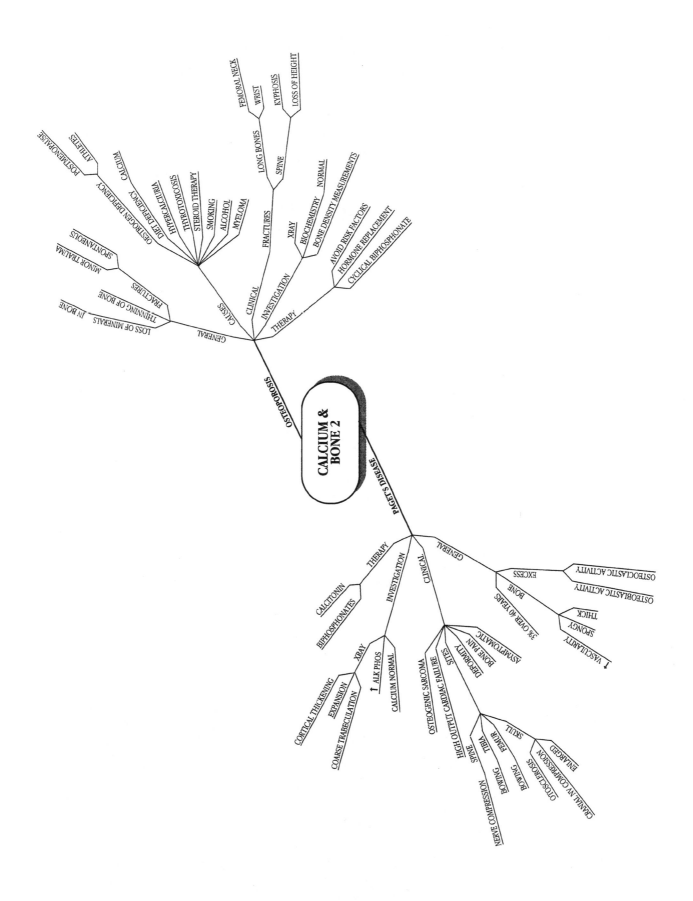

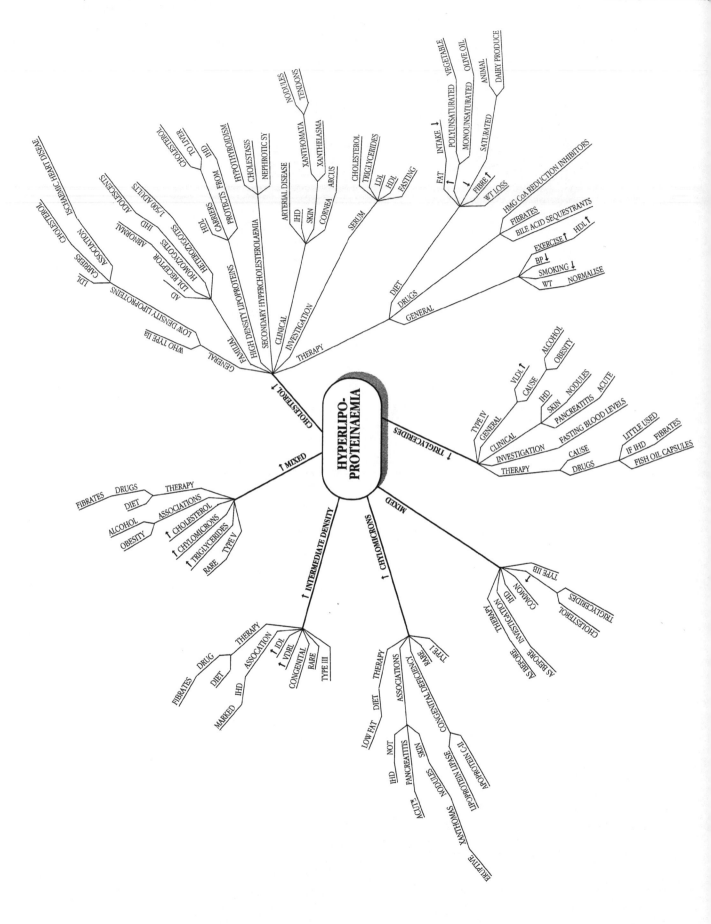

Endocrine

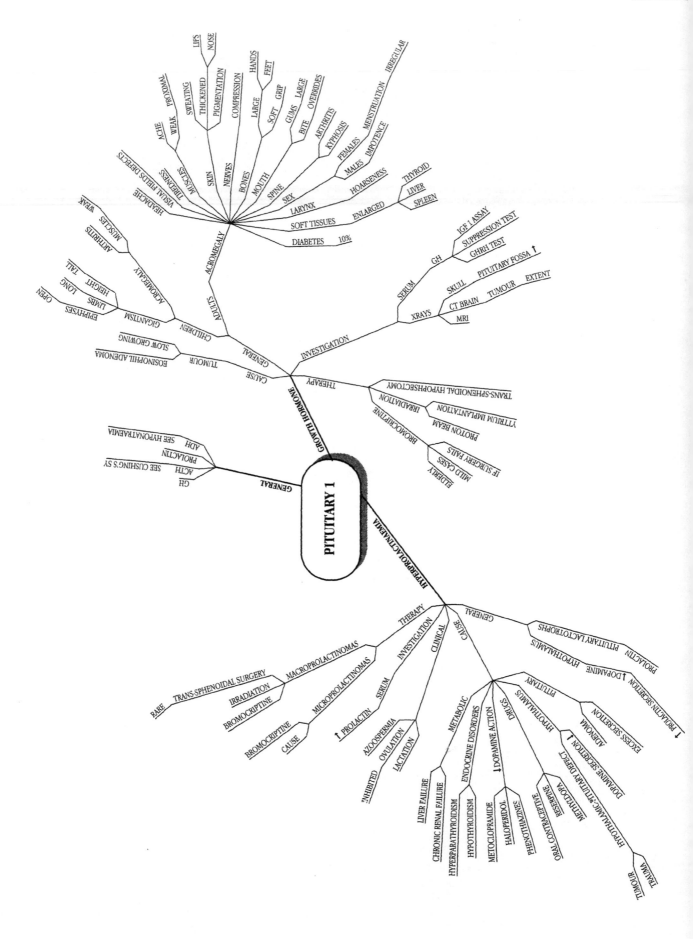

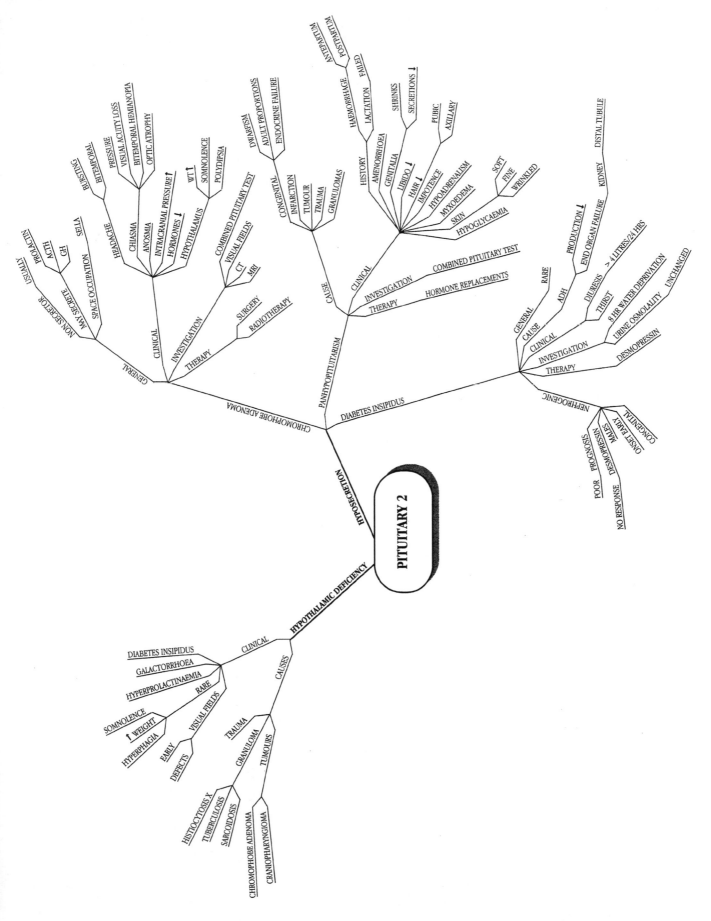

PITUITARY 2

HYPOSECRETION

CHROMOPHOBE ADENOMA

GENERAL
- NON SECRETOR
- MAY SECRETE
  - USUALLY
  - PROLACTIN
  - ACTH
  - GH
- SPACE OCCUPATION
  - SELLA
  - HEADACHE
  - CHIASMA
    - BURSTING
    - BITEMPORAL
    - PRESSURE
    - VISUAL ACUITY LOSS
    - BITEMPORAL HEMIANOPIA
    - OPTIC ATROPHY
  - ANOSMIA
  - INTRACRANIAL PRESSURE ↑
  - HORMONES ↓
  - HYPOTHALAMUS
    - WT ↑
    - SOMNOLENCE
    - POLYDIPSIA

CLINICAL

INVESTIGATION
- COMBINED PITUITARY TEST
- VISUAL FIELDS
- CT
- MRI

THERAPY
- SURGERY
- RADIOTHERAPY

PANHYPOPITUITARISM

CAUSE
- DWARFISM
- ADULT PROPORTIONS
- ENDOCRINE FAILURE
- CONGENITAL
- INFARCTION
- TUMOUR
- TRAUMA
- GRANULOMAS

CLINICAL
- HISTORY
  - HAEMORRHAGE
    - ANTEPARTUM
    - POSTPARTUM
  - LACTATION
    - FAILED
  - SHRINKS
  - SECRETIONS ↓
- AMENORRHOEA
- GENITALIA
- LIBIDO ↓
- HAIR ↓
  - PUBIC
  - AXILLARY
- IMPOTENCE
- HYPOADRENALISM
- MYXOEDEMA
- SKIN
  - SOFT
  - FINE
  - WRINKLED
- HYPOGLYCAEMIA

INVESTIGATION
- COMBINED PITUITARY TEST

THERAPY
- HORMONE REPLACEMENTS

DIABETES INSIPIDUS

GENERAL
- RARE
- ADH
  - PRODUCTION ↓
  - END ORGAN FAILURE
    - KIDNEY
    - DISTAL TUBULE

CAUSE

CLINICAL
- DIURESIS
  - > 4 LITRES/24 HRS
- THIRST

INVESTIGATION
- 8 HR WATER DEPRIVATION
- URINE OSMOLALITY
  - UNCHANGED
- DESMOPRESSIN

THERAPY
- DESMOPRESSIN

NEPHROGENIC
- CONGENITAL
- ONSET EARLY
- MALES
- DESMOPRESSIN
- PROGNOSIS
  - POOR
  - NO RESPONSE

HYPOTHALAMIC DEFICIENCY

CLINICAL
- DIABETES INSIPIDUS
- GALACTORRHOEA
- HYPERPROLACTINAEMIA
- RARE
  - SOMNOLENCE
  - ↑ WEIGHT
  - HYPERPHAGIA
  - VISUAL FIELDS
    - EARLY
    - DEFECTS

CAUSES
- TRAUMA
- GRANULOMA
  - HISTIOCYTOSIS X
  - TUBERCULOSIS
  - SARCOIDOSIS
- TUMOURS
  - CHROMOPHOBE ADENOMA
  - CRANIOPHARYNGIOMA

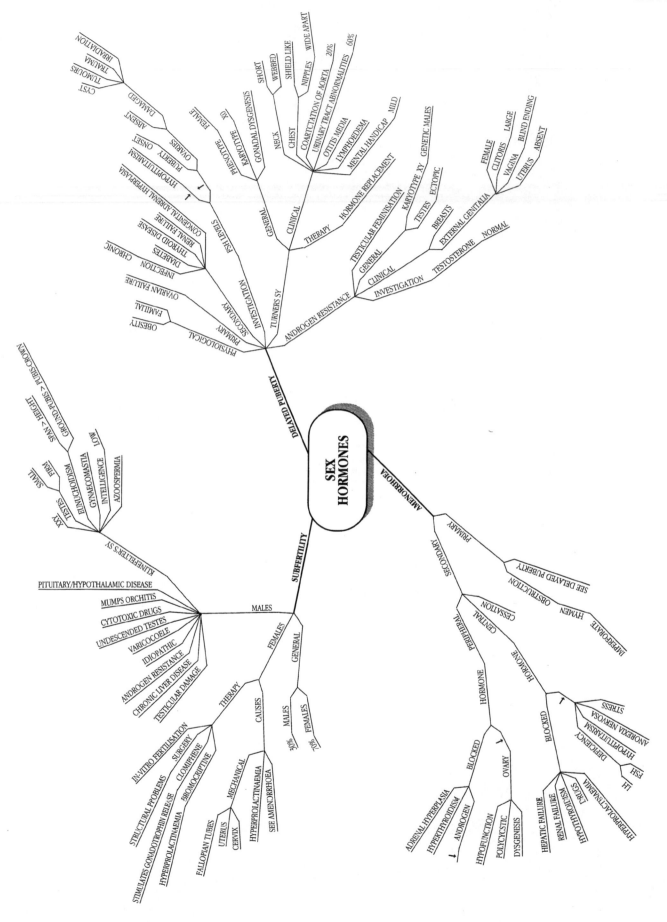

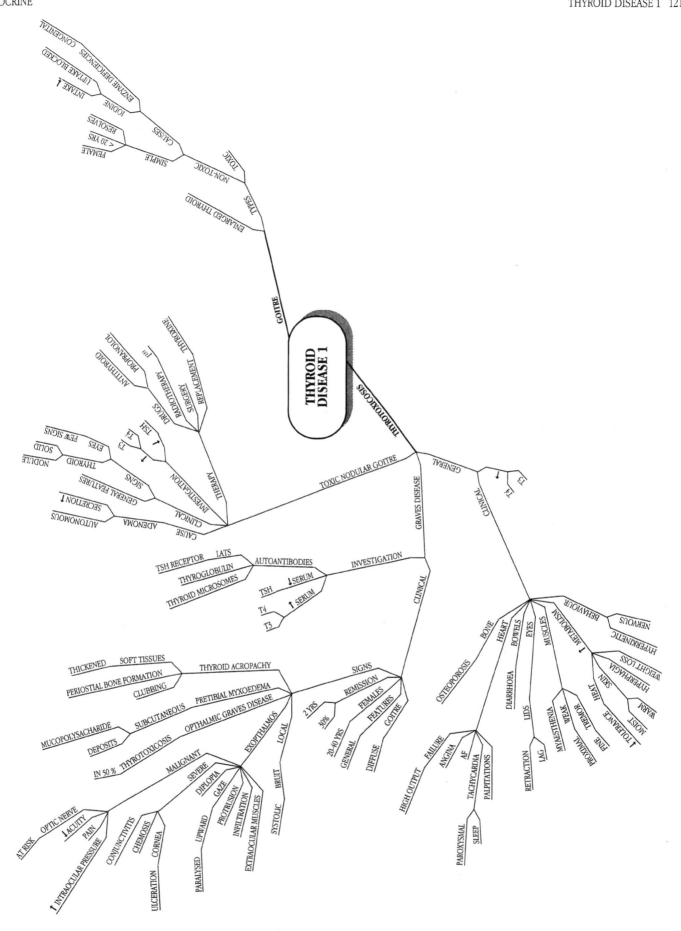

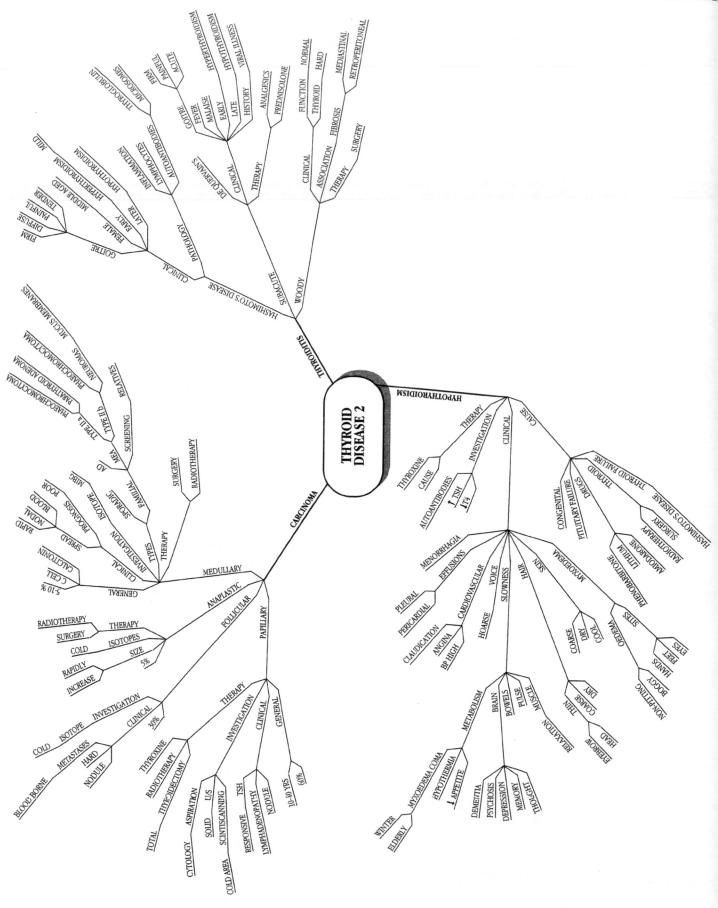

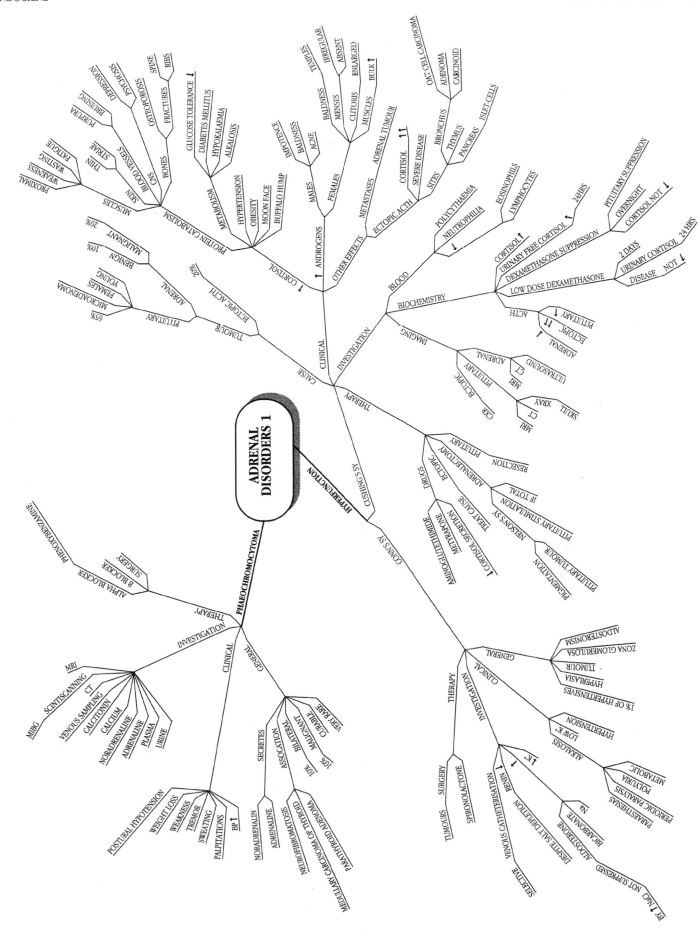

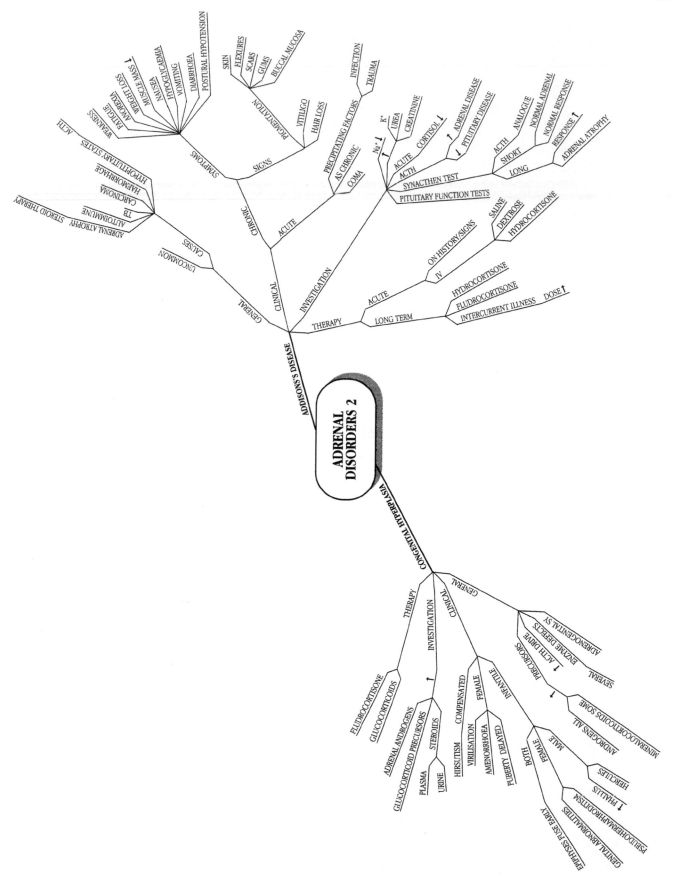

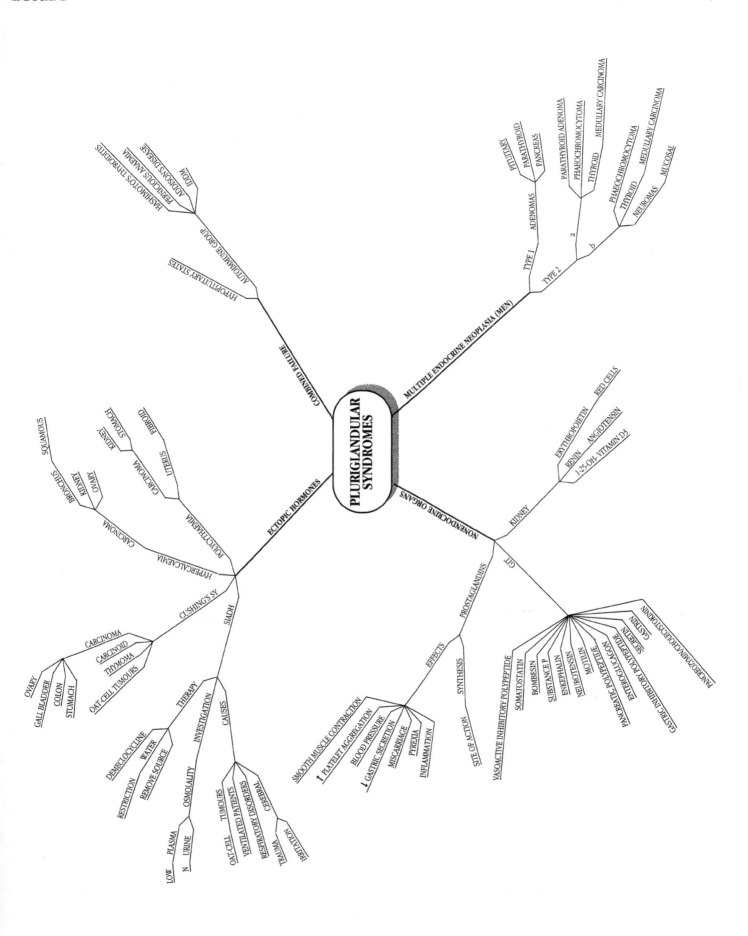

Connective tissues and joints

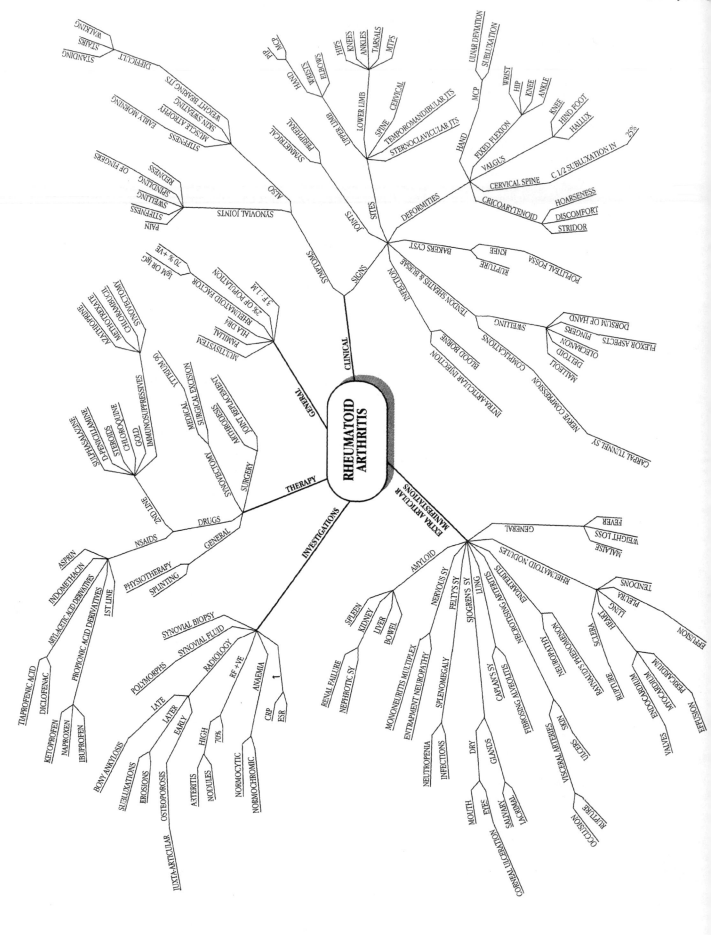

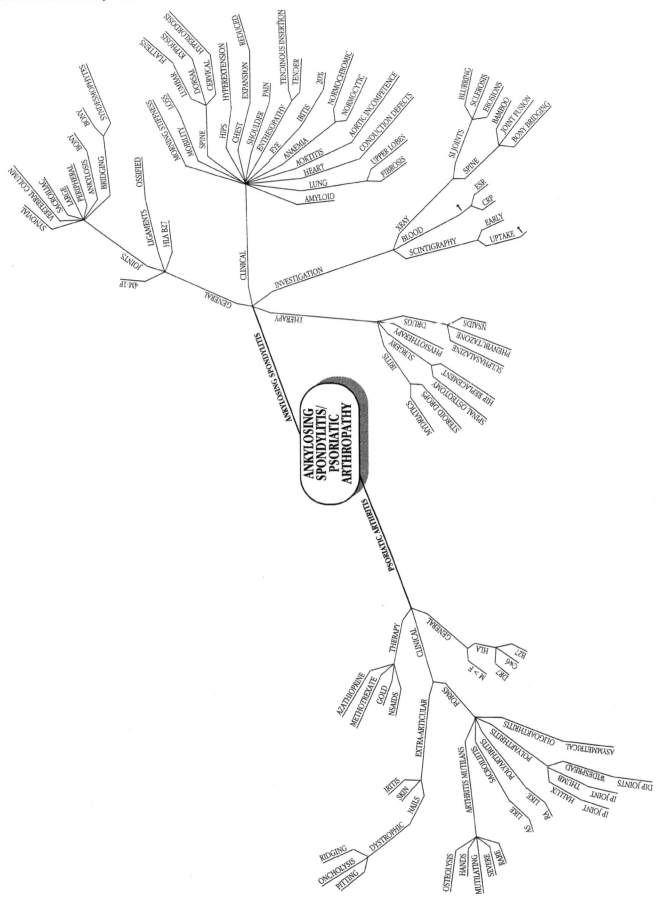

ANKYLOSING SPONDYLITIS/PSORIATIC ARTHROPATHY

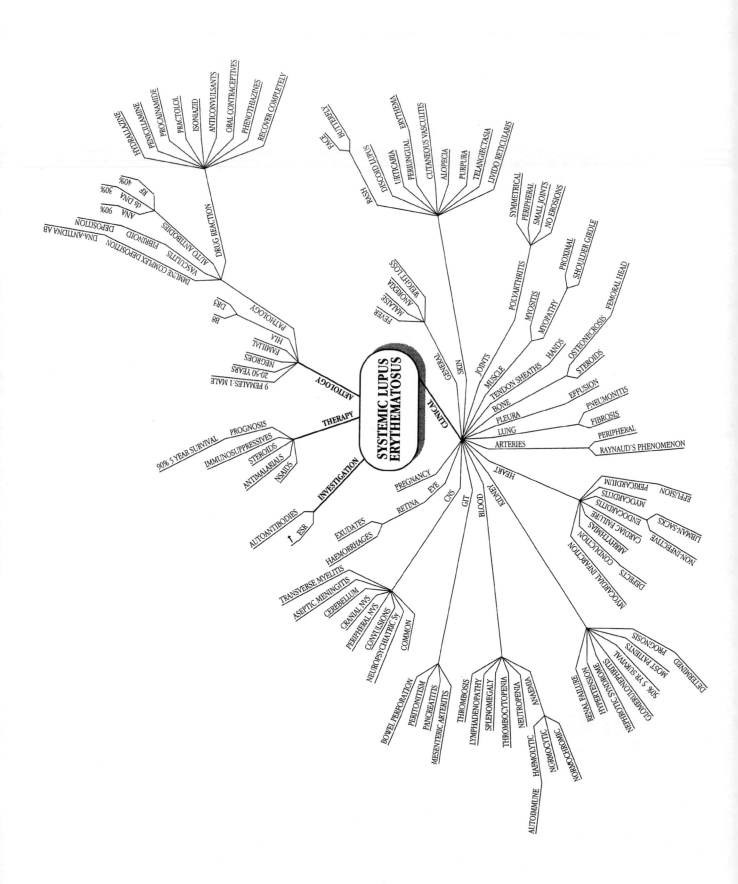

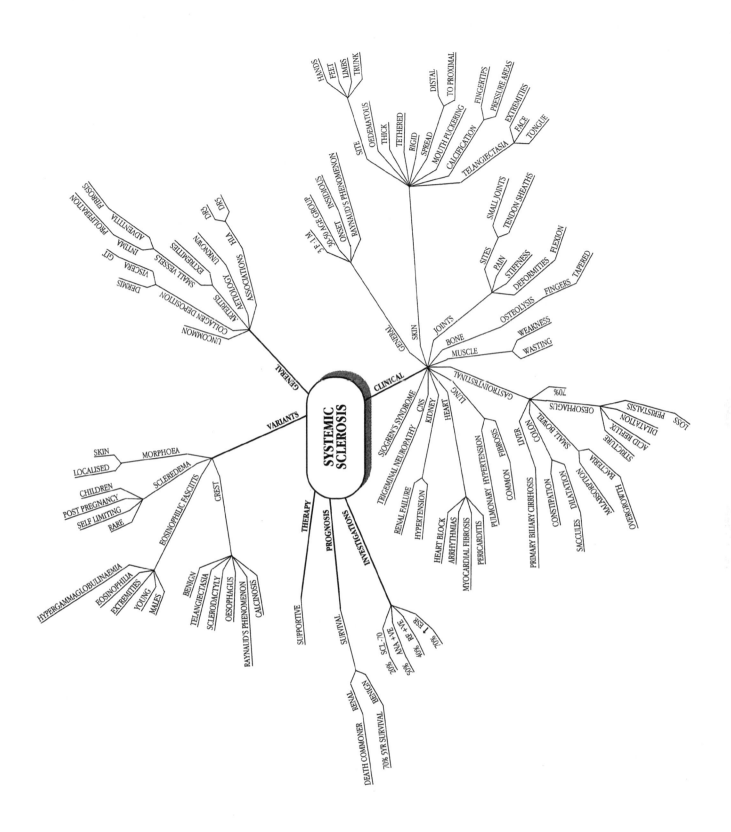

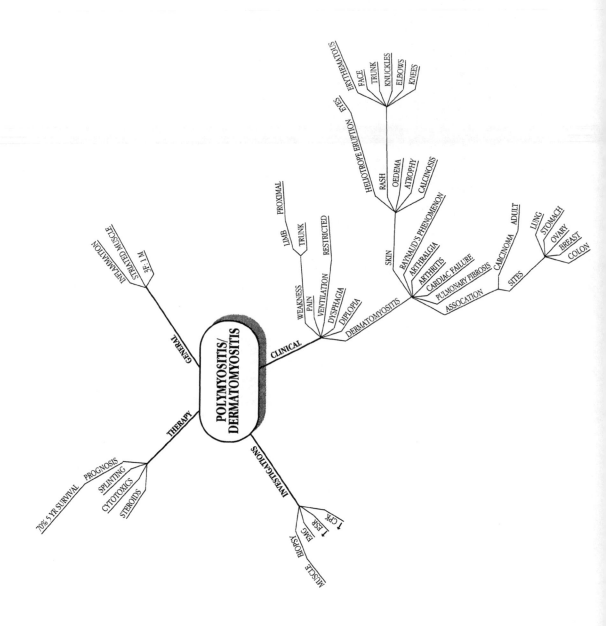

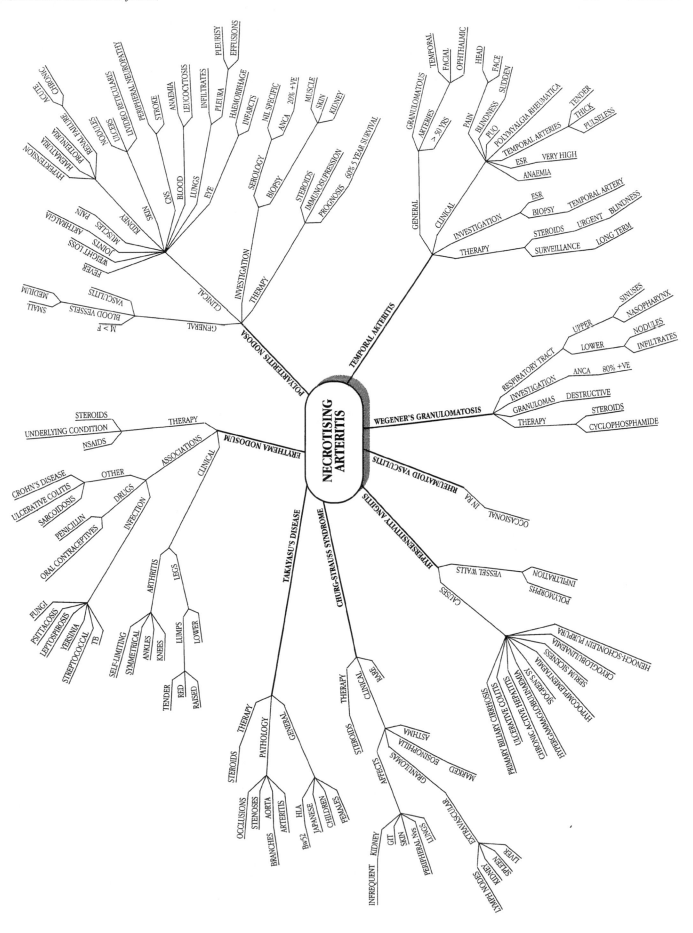

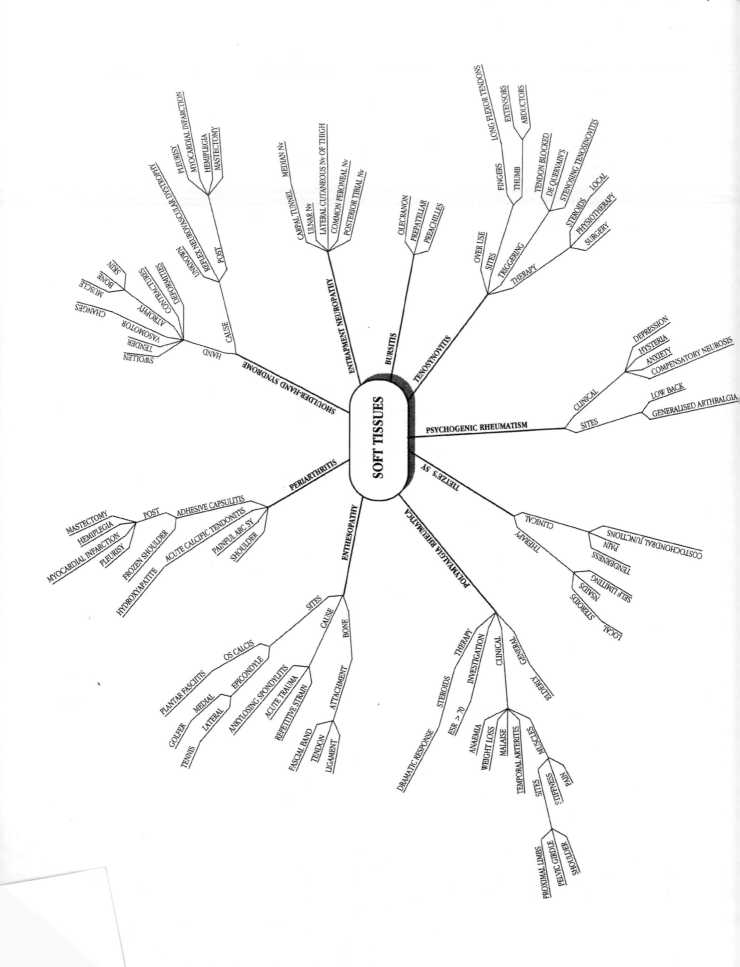

SOFT TISSUES

ENTRAPMENT NEUROPATHY
- CARPAL TUNNEL — MEDIAN Nv
- ULNAR Nv
- LATERAL CUTANEOUS Nv OF THIGH
- COMMON PERONEAL Nv
- POSTERIOR TIBIAL Nv

BURSITIS
- OLECRANON
- PREPATELLAR
- PREACHILLES

TENOSYNOVITIS
- OVER USE
- SITES
  - FINGERS
  - THUMB
  - TENDON BLOCKED — DE QUERVAIN'S — STENOSING TENOSINOVITIS
    - LONG FLEXOR TENDONS
    - EXTENSORS
    - ABDUCTORS
- TRIGGERING
- THERAPY
  - STEROIDS — LOCAL
  - PHYSIOTHERAPY
  - SURGERY

PSYCHOGENIC RHEUMATISM
- CLINICAL
  - DEPRESSION
  - HYSTERIA
  - ANXIETY
  - COMPENSATORY NEUROSIS
- SITES
  - LOW BACK
  - GENERALISED ARTHRALGIA

TIETZE'S SY
- CLINICAL
  - PAIN
  - TENDERNESS
  - COSTOCHONDRAL JUNCTIONS
- THERAPY
  - SELF LIMITING
  - NSAIDS
  - STEROIDS — LOCAL

POLYMYALGIA RHEUMATICA
- THERAPY
  - STEROIDS — DRAMATIC RESPONSE
- INVESTIGATION — ESR > 70
- CLINICAL
  - GENERAL
    - ELDERLY
    - ANAEMIA
    - WEIGHT LOSS
    - MALAISE
    - TEMPORAL ARTERITIS
  - MUSCLES
    - SITES
      - PROXIMAL LIMBS
      - PELVIC GIRDLE
      - SHOULDER
    - STIFFNESS
    - PAIN

ENTHESOPATHY
- SITES
  - PLANTAR FASCIITIS — OS CALCIS
  - GOLFER — MEDIAL
  - TENNIS — LATERAL
  - EPICONDYLE
  - ANKYLOSING SPONDYLITIS
- CAUSE
  - ACUTE TRAUMA
  - REPETITIVE STRAIN
  - BONE
  - ATTACHMENT
    - FASCIAL BAND
    - TENDON
    - LIGAMENT

PERIARTHRITIS
- ADHESIVE CAPSULITIS
  - POST
    - MASTECTOMY
    - HEMIPLEGIA
    - MYOCARDIAL INFARCTION
    - PLEURISY
  - FROZEN SHOULDER
- ACUTE CALCIFIC TENDONITIS
  - HYDROXYAPATITE
- PAINFUL ARC SY — SHOULDER

SHOULDER-HAND SYNDROME
- HAND
  - SWOLLEN
  - TENDER
  - VASOMOTOR — CHANGES
  - ATROPHY
    - MUSCLE
    - BONE
    - SKIN
  - CONTRACTURES
  - DEFORMITIES
- CAUSE
  - UNKNOWN
  - REFLEX NEUROVASCULAR DYSTROPHY
  - POST
    - PLEURISY
    - MYOCARDIAL INFARCTION
    - HEMIPLEGIA
    - MASTECTOMY

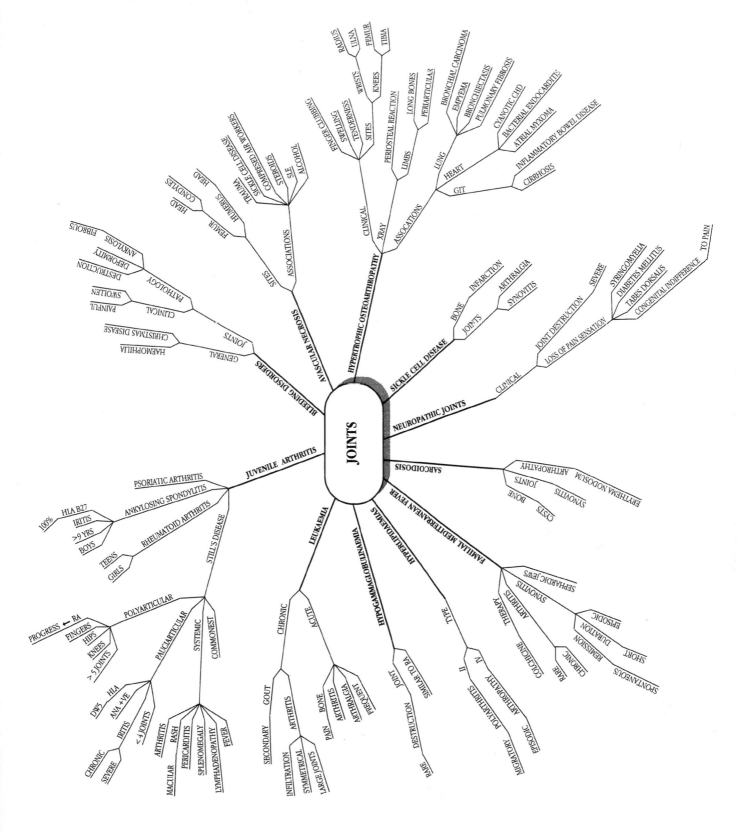

JOINTS

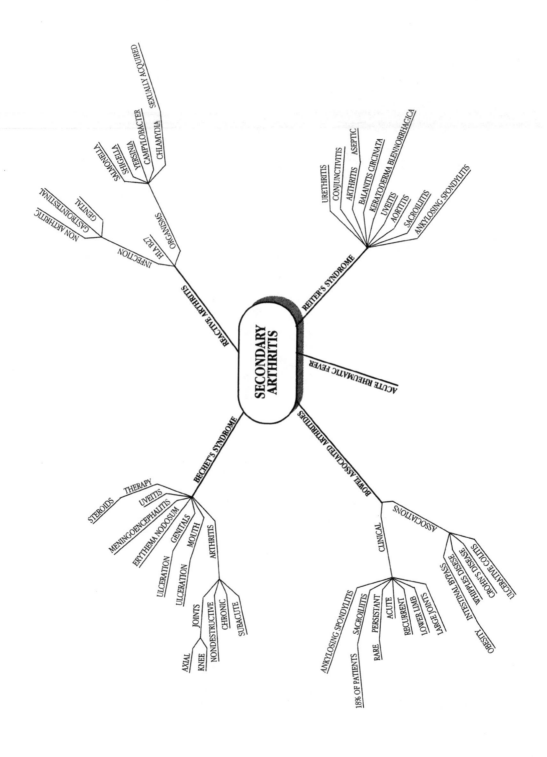

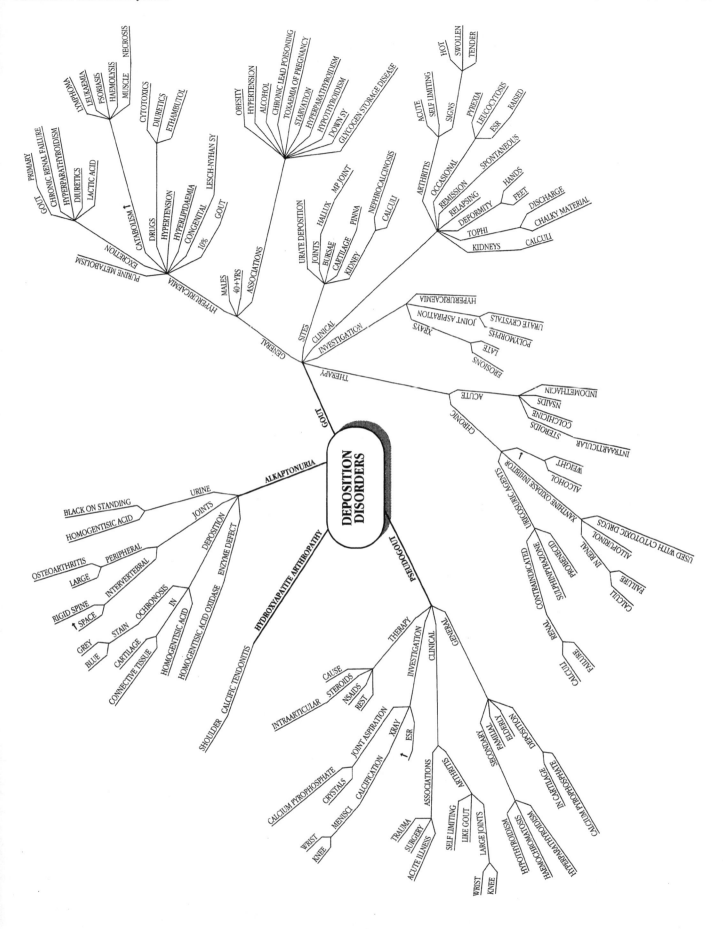

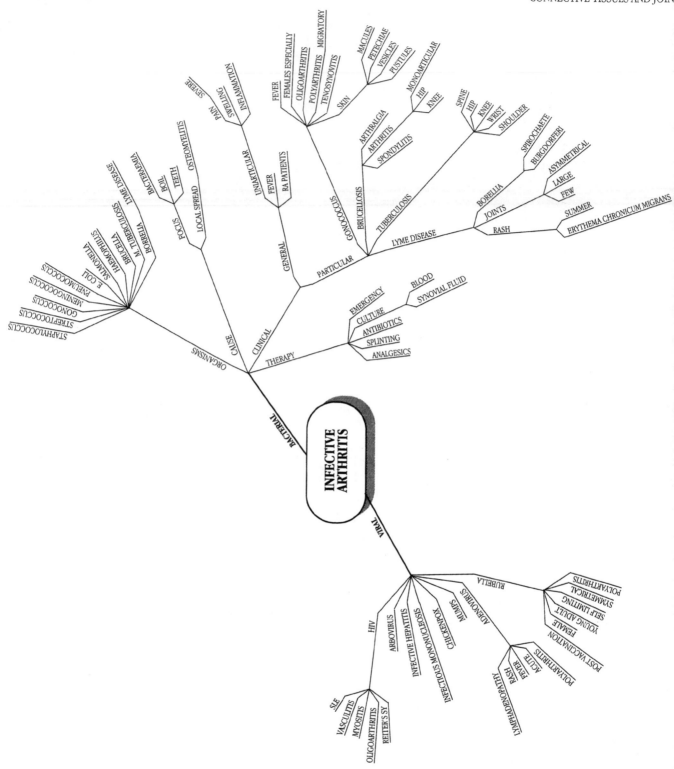

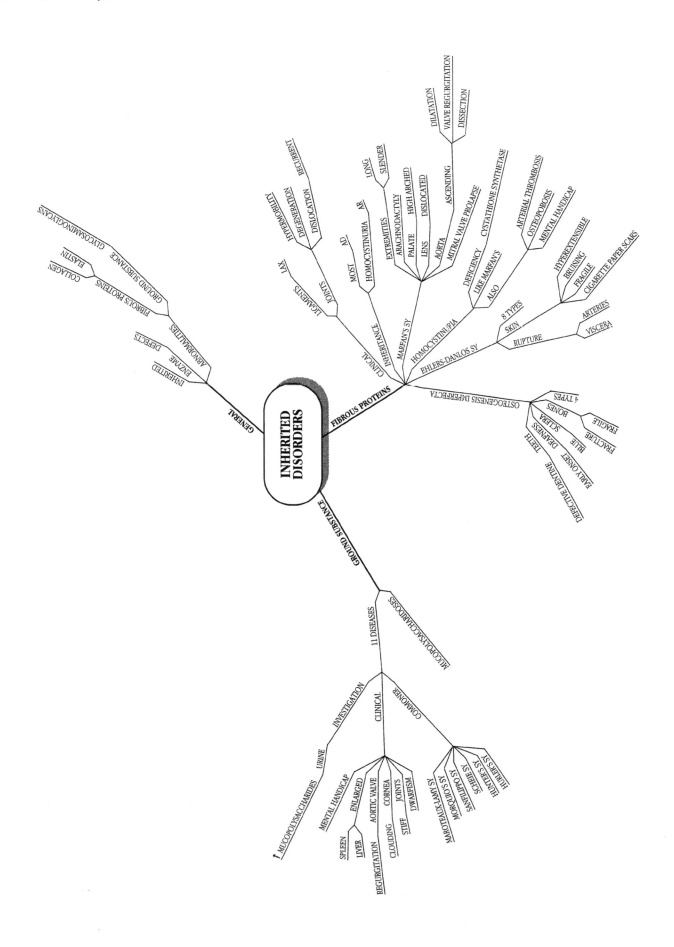

INHERITED DISORDERS

GENERAL

INHERITED — ENZYME — ABNORMALITIES — FIBROUS PROTEINS — COLLAGEN
ELASTIN
DEFECTS — GROUND SUBSTANCE — GLYCOSAMINOGLYCANS

FIBROUS PROTEINS

CLINICAL — INHERITANCE
LAX — LIGAMENTS — JOINTS — HYPERMOBILITY — DEGENERATION — DISLOCATION — RECURRENT
MOST — AD
HOMOCYSTINURIA — AR

MARFAN'S SY
EXTREMITIES — ARACHNODACTYLY — LONG
PALATE — HIGH ARCHED
LENS — DISLOCATED — SLENDER
AORTA — ASCENDING — DILATATION
MITRAL VALVE PROLAPSE — VALVE REGURGITATION
DISSECTION

HOMOCYSTINURIA
DEFICIENCY — CYSTATHIONE SYNTHETASE
LIKE MARFAN'S
ALSO — ARTERIAL THROMBOSIS
OSTEOPOROSIS
MENTAL HANDICAP

EHLERS-DANLOS SY
8 TYPES
SKIN — HYPEREXTENSIBLE
BRUISING
FRAGILE
CIGARETTE PAPER SCARS
RUPTURE — ARTERIES
VISCERA

OSTEOGENESIS IMPERFECTA
4 TYPES
BONES — FRAGILE
FRACTURE
SCLERA — BLUE
DEAFNESS — EARLY ONSET
TEETH — DEFECTIVE DENTINE

GROUND SUBSTANCE

MUCOPOLYSACCHARIDOSIS
11 DISEASES
INVESTIGATION — URINE — ↑ MUCOPOLYSACCHARIDES
CLINICAL
MENTAL HANDICAP
SPLEEN — ENLARGED
LIVER
AORTIC VALVE — REGURGITATION
CORNEA — CLOUDING
JOINTS — STIFF
DWARFISM
COMMONER
MAROTEAUX-LAMY SY
MORQUIO'S SY
SANFILIPPO SY
SCHEIE SY
HUNTER'S SY
HURLER'S SY

Infectious diseases

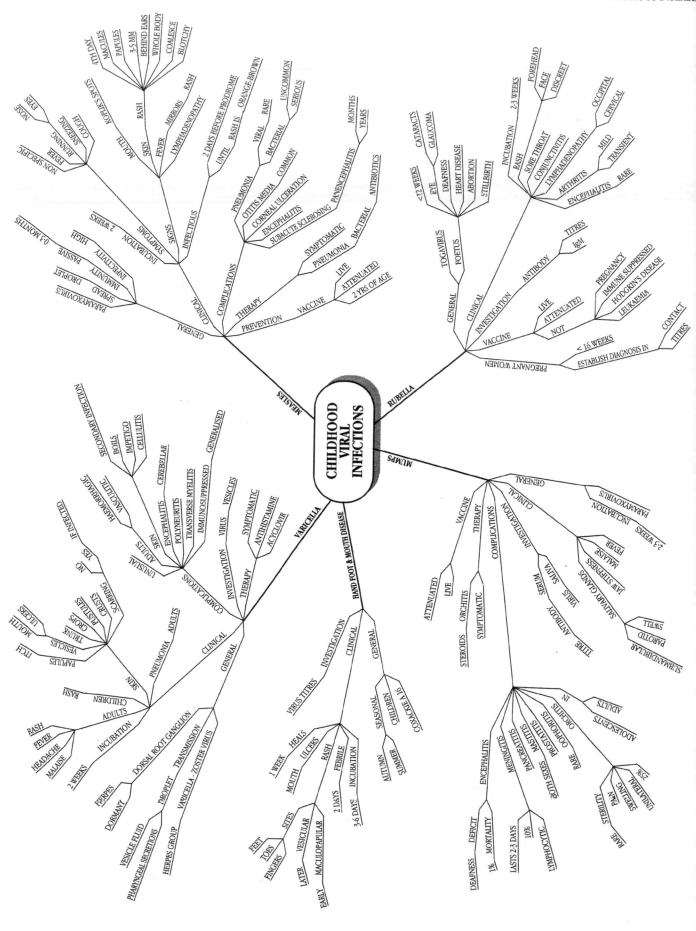

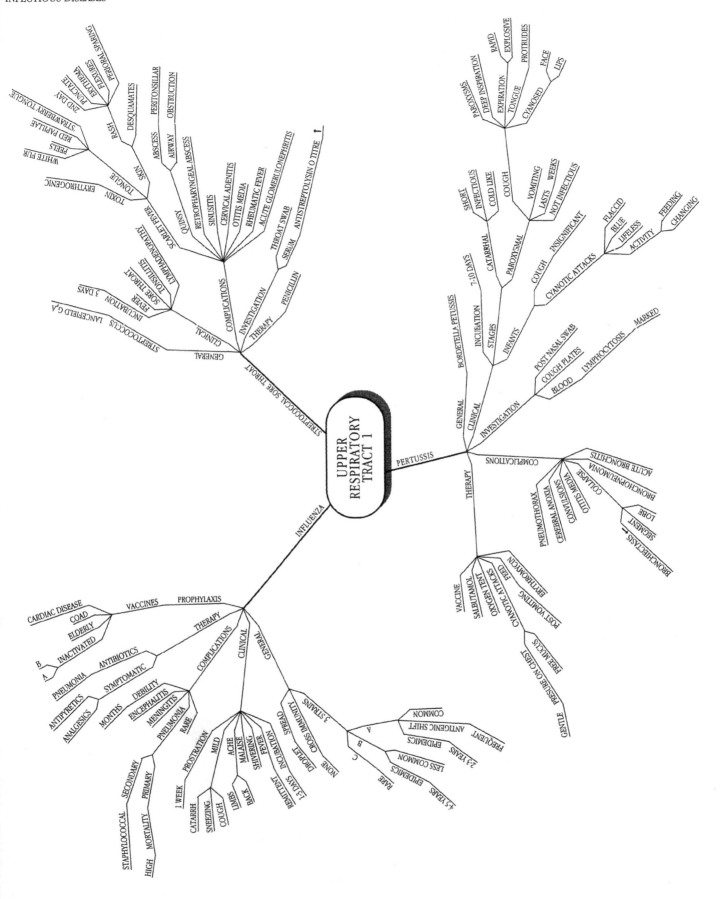

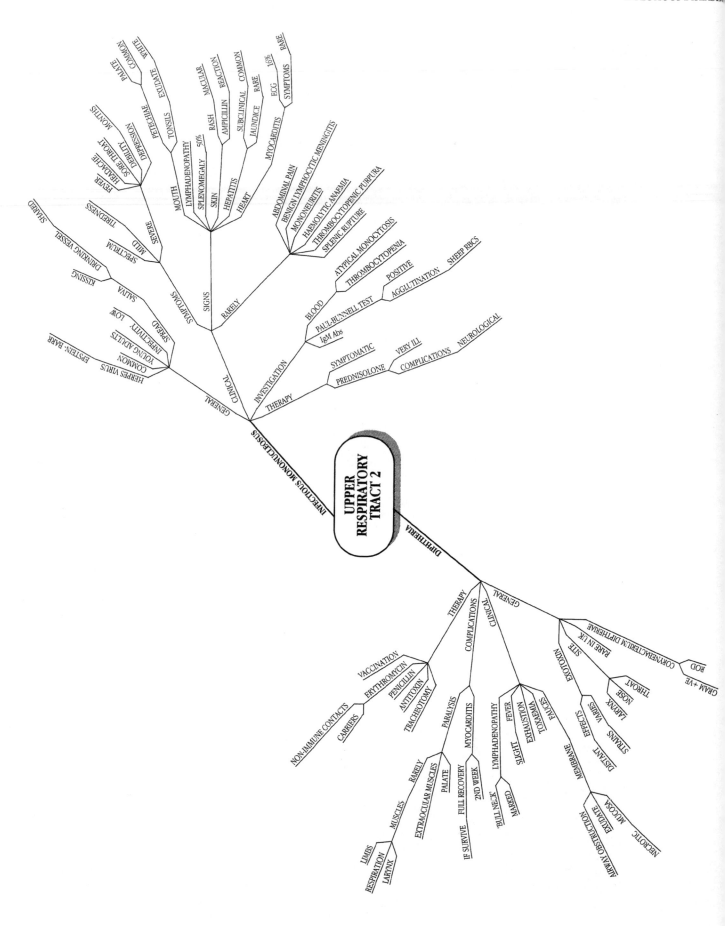

UPPER RESPIRATORY TRACT 2

INFECTIOUS MONONUCLEOSIS

- GENERAL
  - CLINICAL
    - HERPES VIRUS: EPSTEIN-BARR
    - SPREAD
      - COMMON: YOUNG ADULTS
      - INFECTIVITY: LOW
      - SALIVA
        - KISSING
        - DRINKING VESSEL
    - SYMPTOMS
      - SPECTRUM
        - MILD
        - SEVERE
          - TIREDNESS: SHARED
          - FEVER
          - HEADACHE
          - SORE THROAT
          - DEBILITY: MONTHS
          - DEPRESSION
    - SIGNS
      - MOUTH
        - TONSILS
          - EXUDATE
          - PETECHIAE
        - PALATE: COMMON, WHITE
      - LYMPHADENOPATHY
      - SPLENOMEGALY 50%
      - SKIN
        - RASH: MACULAR
        - AMPICILLIN REACTION: COMMON
      - HEPATITIS
        - SUBCLINICAL
        - JAUNDICE: RARE
      - HEART
        - MYOCARDITIS
          - ECG 16%
          - SYMPTOMS: RARE
      - RARELY
        - ABDOMINAL PAIN
        - BENIGN LYMPHOCYTIC MENINGITIS
        - MONONEURITIS
        - HAEMOLYTIC ANAEMIA
        - THROMBOCYTOPENIC PURPURA
        - SPLENIC RUPTURE
  - INVESTIGATION
    - BLOOD
      - ATYPICAL MONOCYTOSIS
      - THROMBOCYTOPENIA
    - PAUL-BUNNELL TEST
      - IgM Abs
      - AGGLUTINATION: POSITIVE
      - SHEEP RBCS
  - THERAPY
    - SYMPTOMATIC
    - PREDNISOLONE
      - VERY ILL
      - COMPLICATIONS
      - NEUROLOGICAL

DIPHTHERIA

- GENERAL
  - CORYNEBACTERIUM DIPHTHERIAE
    - RARE IN UK
    - GRAM +VE
    - ROD
  - CLINICAL
    - SITE
      - THROAT
      - NOSE
      - LARYNX
    - EXOTOXIN
      - STRAINS: VARIES
      - EFFECTS
        - DISTANT
        - MEMBRANE
          - EXUDATE
          - NECROTIC MUCOSA
          - AIRWAY OBSTRUCTION
    - FAUCES
      - TOXAEMIA
      - EXHAUSTION
      - FEVER: SLIGHT
      - LYMPHADENOPATHY
        - MARKED
        - "BULL NECK"
  - COMPLICATIONS
    - MYOCARDITIS
      - 2ND WEEK
      - FULL RECOVERY: IF SURVIVE
    - PARALYSIS
      - PALATE
      - EXTRAOCULAR MUSCLES
      - RARELY
        - MUSCLES
          - LIMBS
          - RESPIRATION
          - LARYNX
- THERAPY
  - TRACHEOTOMY
  - ANTITOXIN
  - PENICILLIN
  - ERYTHROMYCIN
  - VACCINATION
  - CARRIERS
  - NON-IMMUNE CONTACTS

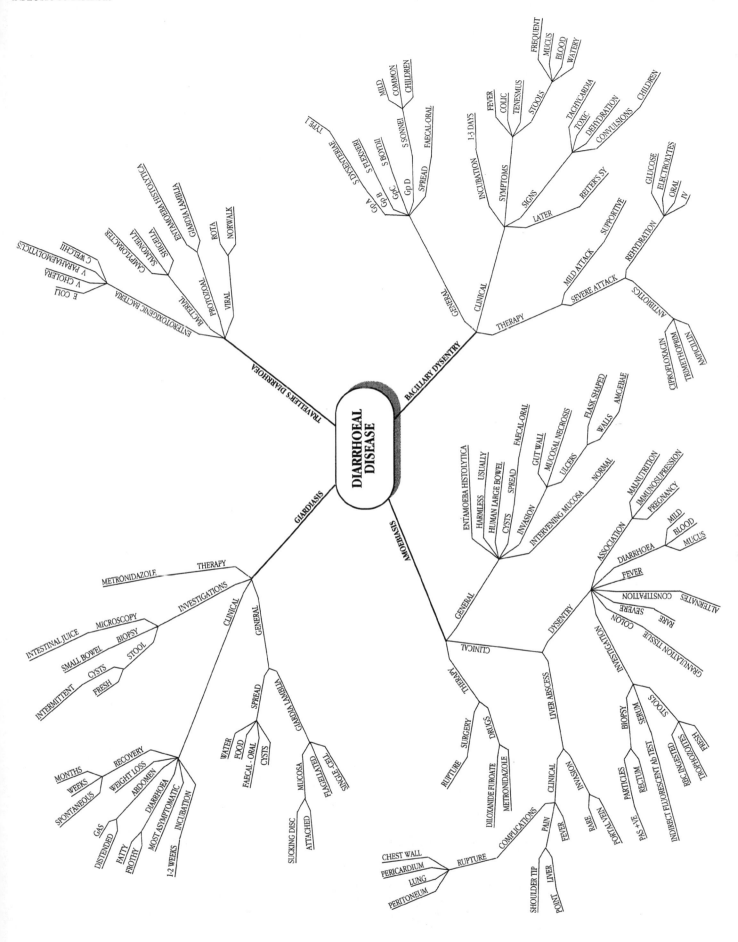

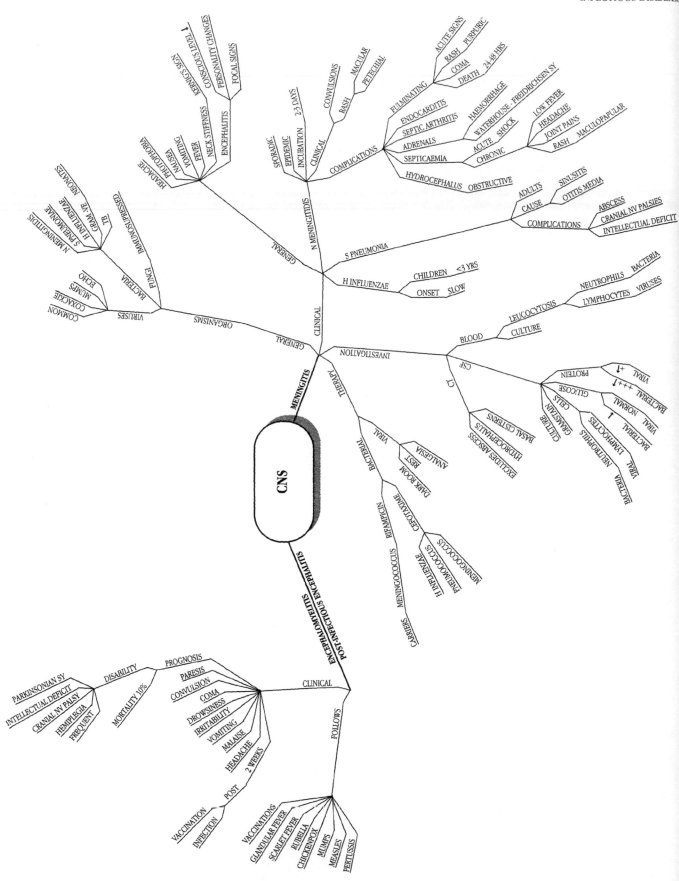

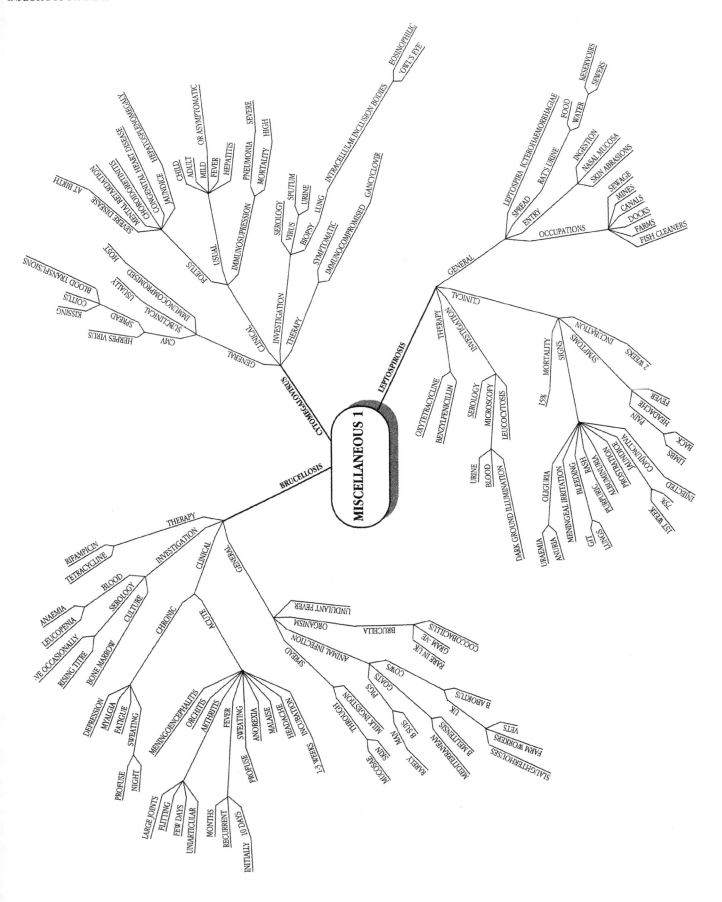

MISCELLANEOUS 1

CYTOMEGALOVIRUS

LEPTOSPIROSIS

BRUCELLOSIS

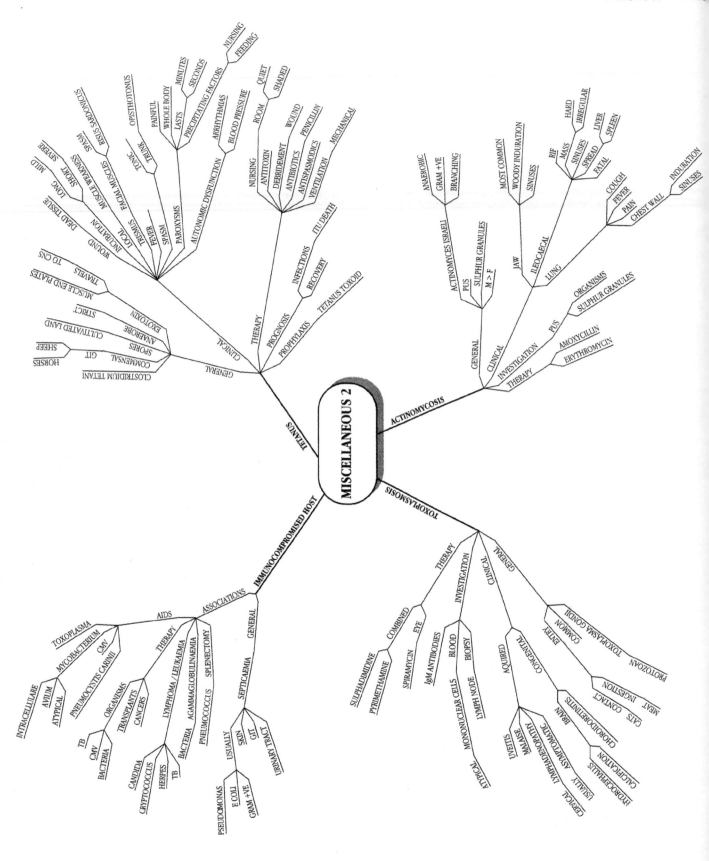

MISCELLANEOUS 2

TETANUS

GENERAL

CLOSTRIDIUM TETANI — GIT — COMMENSAL
— HORSES
— SHEEP
SPORES — CULTIVATED LAND
ANAEROBE — STRICT
EXOTOXIN — MUSCLE END PLATES
— TRAVELS — TO CNS

CLINICAL
WOUND — INCUBATION — DEAD TISSUE — MILD
— LONG — SHORT — SEVERE
FEVER
SPASM — TRISMUS — LOCAL
— FACIAL MUSCLES
MUSCLE WEAKNESS
TRUNK
TONIC — RISUS SARDONICUS
— OPISTHOTONUS
PAROXYSMS — PAINFUL
— WHOLE BODY
— LASTS — MINUTES
— SECONDS
PRECIPITATING FACTORS — NURSING
— FEEDING
AUTONOMIC DYSFUNCTION — ARRHYTHMIAS
— BLOOD PRESSURE

THERAPY — NURSING — ROOM — QUIET
— SHADED
ANTITOXIN
DEBRIDEMENT — WOUND
ANTIBIOTICS — PENICILLIN
ANTISPASMODICS
VENTILATION — MECHANICAL

PROGNOSIS — INFECTIONS — ITU DEATH
— RECOVERY
PROPHYLAXIS — TETANUS TOXOID

ACTINOMYCOSIS

GENERAL — ACTINOMYCES ISRAELI — ANAEROBIC
— GRAM +VE
— BRANCHING
SULPHUR GRANULES — PUS
— M > F
WOODY INDURATION — MOST COMMON
SINUSES

CLINICAL — JAW
ILEOCAECAL — RIF — MASS — HARD
— IRREGULAR
SINUSES — LIVER
— SPREAD — SPLEEN
— FATAL
LUNG — COUGH
— FEVER
— PAIN — CHEST WALL — INDURATION
— SINUSES

INVESTIGATION — PUS — ORGANISMS
— SULPHUR GRANULES

THERAPY — AMOXYCILLIN
— ERYTHROMYCIN

TOXOPLASMOSIS

GENERAL — TOXOPLASMA GONDII — PROTOZOAN
— COMMON
ENTRY — MEAT INGESTION
— CATS CONTACT

CLINICAL — CONGENITAL — HYDROCEPHALUS
— CHORIORETINITIS
— BRAIN CALCIFICATION
ACQUIRED — USUALLY ASYMPTOMATIC
— CERVICAL LYMPHADENOPATHY
— MALAISE
— UVEITIS

INVESTIGATION — BIOPSY — LYMPH NODE — ATYPICAL MONONUCLEAR CELLS
BLOOD — IgM ANTIBODIES
EYE

THERAPY — COMBINED — SPIRAMYCIN
— PYRIMETHAMINE
— SULPHADIMIDINE

IMMUNOCOMPROMISED HOST

ASSOCIATIONS

AIDS — TOXOPLASMA
— MYCOBACTERIUM — INTRACELLULARE
— AVIUM
— ATYPICAL
— TB
CMV
PNEUMOCYSTIS CARINII
THERAPY — ORGANISMS — CMV
— BACTERIA
— CANDIDA
— CRYPTOCOCCUS
— HERPES
— TB
TRANSPLANTS
CANCERS — LYMPHOMA / LEUKAEMIA
AGAMMAGLOBULINAEMIA — PNEUMOCOCCUS
SPLENECTOMY — BACTERIA

GENERAL — SEPTICAEMIA — USUALLY — SKIN
— GIT — PSEUDOMONAS
— E COLI
— GRAM +VE
— URINARY TRACT

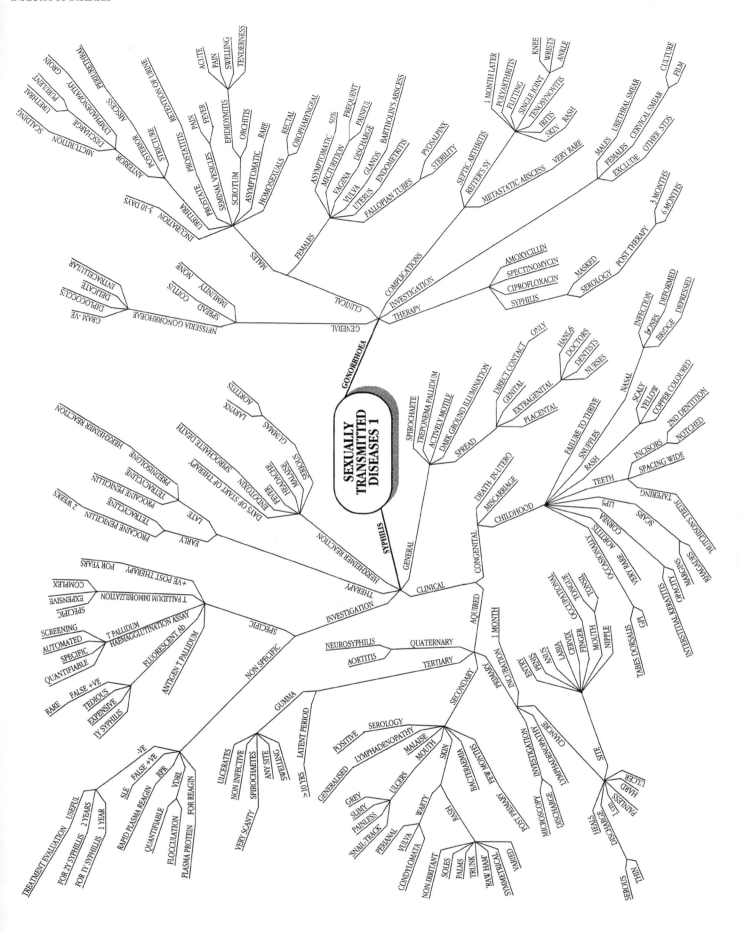

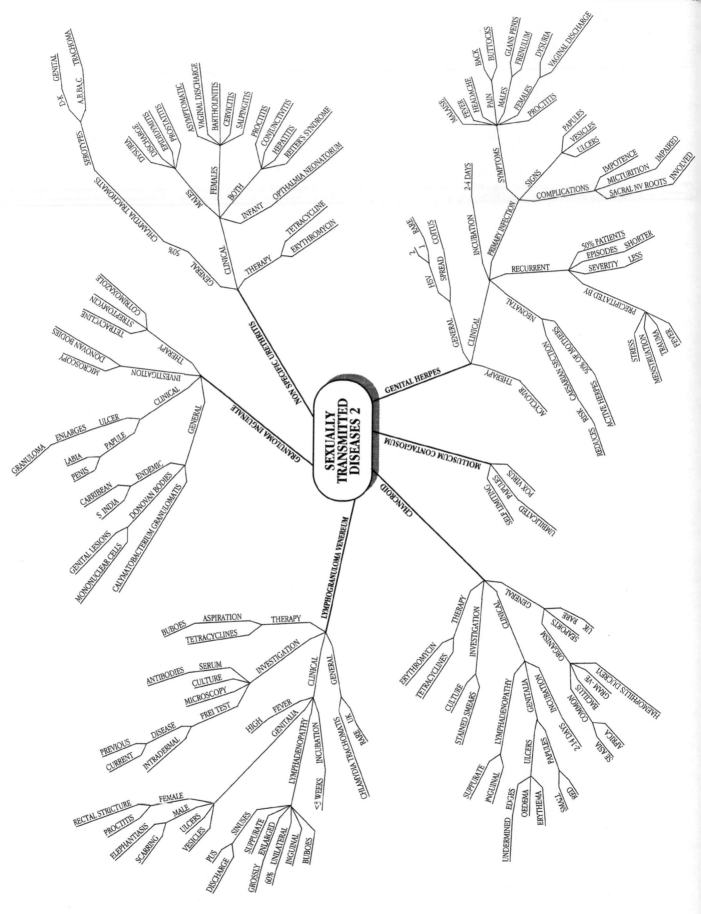

Tropical

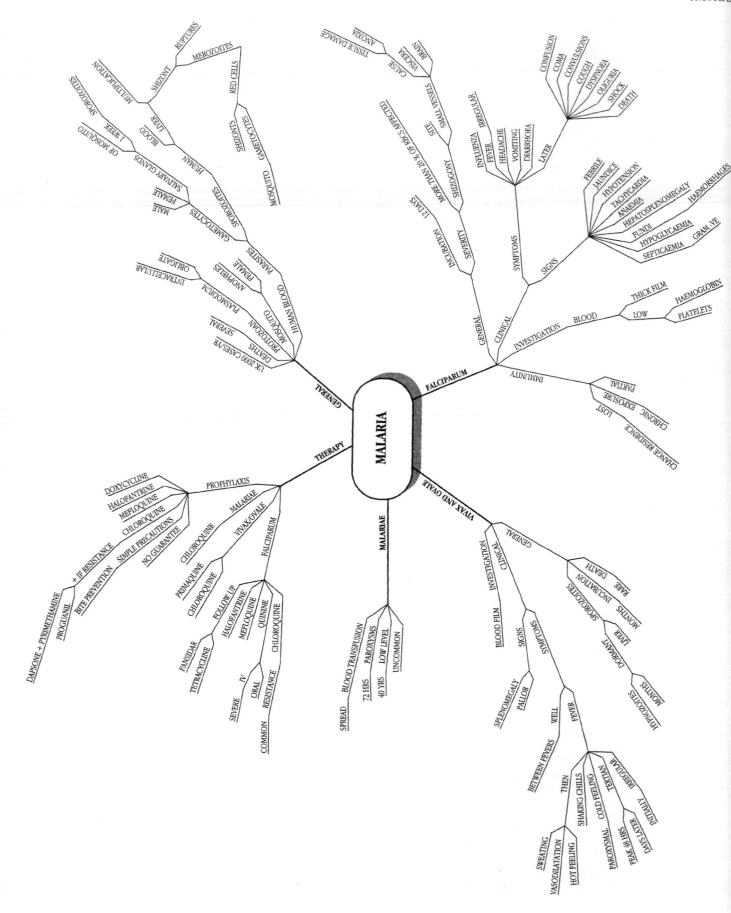

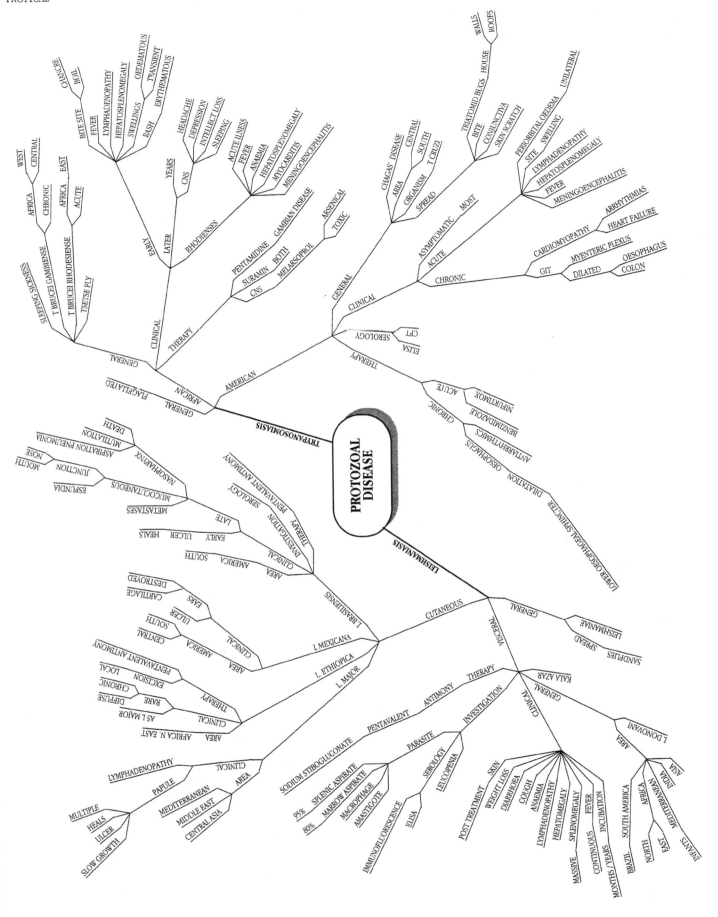

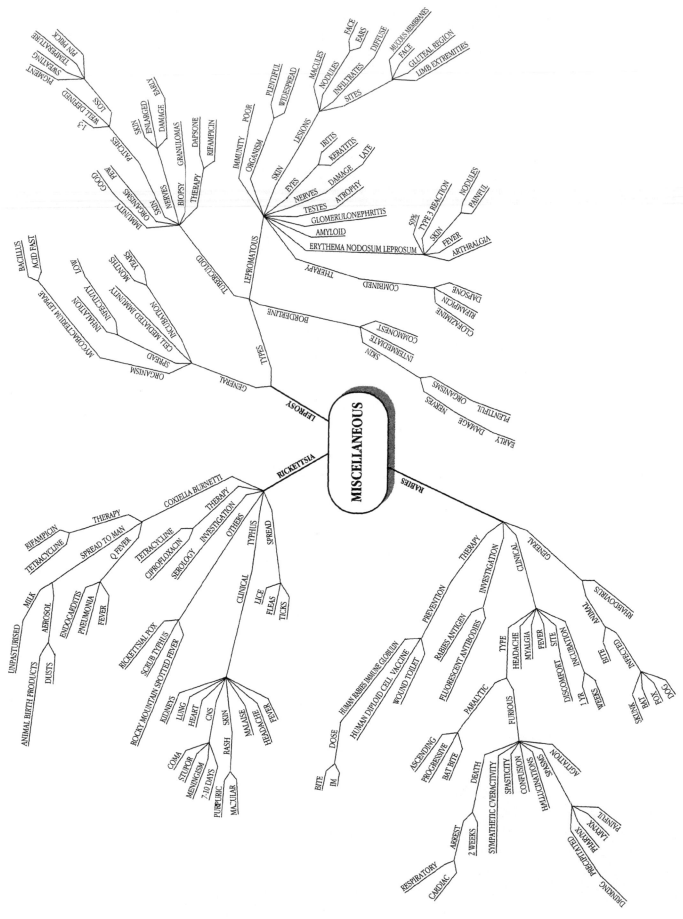

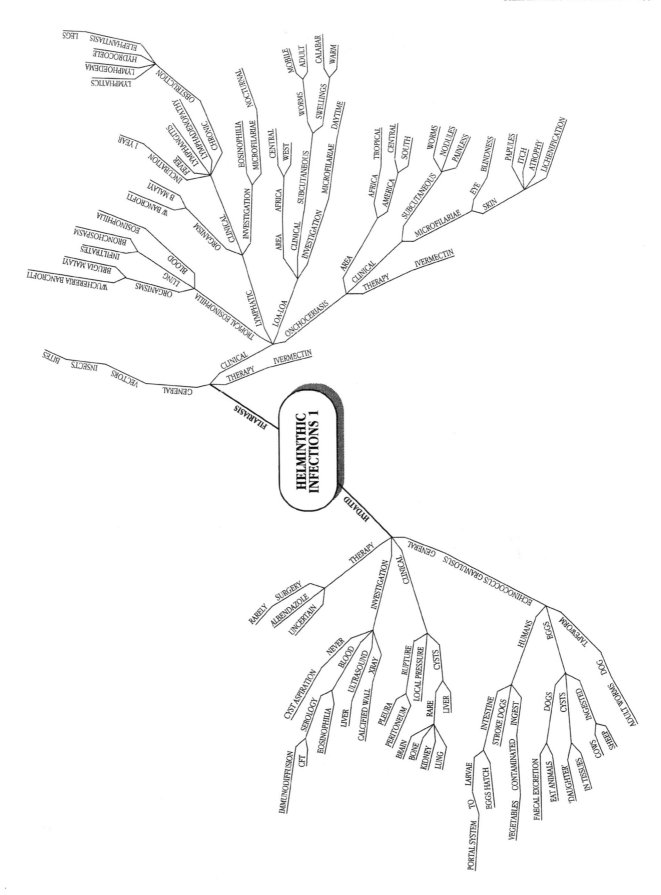

HELMINTHIC INFECTIONS 1

FILARIASIS

GENERAL
- VECTORS — INSECTS — BITES
- CLINICAL
- THERAPY — IVERMECTIN

TROPICAL EOSINOPHILIA
- ORGANISMS
  - WUCHERERIA BANCROFTI
  - BRUGIA MALAYI
- LUNG
  - INFILTRATES
  - BRONCHOSPASM
- BLOOD
  - EOSINOPHILIA

LYMPHATIC
- ORGANISM
  - W BANCROFTI
  - B MALAYI
- CLINICAL
  - INCUBATION — 1 YEAR
  - FEVER
  - LYMPHANGITIS
  - LYMPHADENOPATHY — CHRONIC
  - OBSTRUCTION
    - LYMPHATICS
    - LYMPHOEDEMA
    - HYDROCOELE
    - ELEPHANTIASIS — LEGS
- INVESTIGATION
  - EOSINOPHILIA
  - MICROFILARIAE — NOCTURNAL

LOA-LOA
- AREA — AFRICA
  - CENTRAL
  - WEST
- SUBCUTANEOUS — WORMS
  - MOBILE
  - ADULT
- SWELLINGS — CALABAR — WARM
- CLINICAL
- INVESTIGATION — MICROFILARIAE — DAYTIME

ONCHOCERIASIS
- AREA
  - AFRICA
  - TROPICAL
  - AMERICA
    - CENTRAL
    - SOUTH
- SUBCUTANEOUS — WORMS
  - NODULES
  - PAINLESS
- MICROFILARIAE
  - EYE — BLINDNESS
  - SKIN
    - PAPULES
    - ITCH
    - ATROPHY
    - LICHENIFICATION
- CLINICAL
- THERAPY — IVERMECTIN

HYDATID

ECHINOCOCCUS GRANULOSUS

GENERAL
- TAPEWORM
  - DOG — ADULT WORMS
  - SHEEP
  - COWS — INGESTED — IN TISSUES
  - DOGS — CYSTS — 'DAUGHTER'
  - FAECAL EXCRETION — EAT ANIMALS
  - HUMANS — EGGS
    - INGEST — CONTAMINATED — VEGETABLES
    - STROKE DOGS
    - INTESTINE — EGGS HATCH — LARVAE — TO — PORTAL SYSTEM

CLINICAL
- CYSTS
  - LIVER — RARE
  - LUNG
  - KIDNEY
  - BONE
  - BRAIN
  - PERITONEUM
  - PLEURA
  - LOCAL PRESSURE
  - RUPTURE

INVESTIGATION
- XRAY
  - CALCIFIED WALL
  - LIVER
- ULTRASOUND
- BLOOD
  - EOSINOPHILIA
  - SEROLOGY
    - CFT
    - IMMUNODIFFUSION
- CYST ASPIRATION — NEVER

THERAPY
- SURGERY
- ALBENDAZOLE — UNCERTAIN
- RARELY

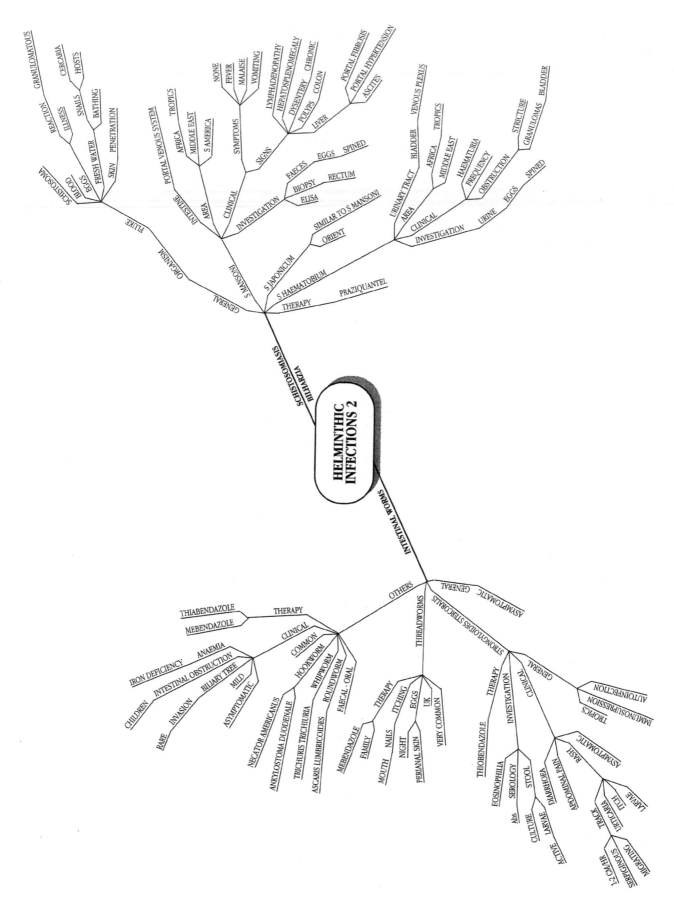

Further reading and information

Buzan T 2003 Use your head. BBC Books

Buzan T 2003 The mind map book. BBC Books

Buzan T 2003 The speed reading book. BBC Books

Haslett C, Chilvers E R, Boon N A, Colledge N R, Hunter J A A 2002 Davidson's principles and practice of medicine, 19th edn. Churchill Livingstone

Longmore J M et al 2001 Oxford handbook of clinical medicine, 5th edn. Oxford University Press

Souhami R L, Moxham J 2002 Textbook of medicine, 4th edn. Churchill Livingstone

For further information on Mind Map books, videos, audio tapes and other products please contact the addresses below for a brochure.

UK HEAD OFFICE

Buzan Centres Ltd.
54 Parkstone Road
Poole
Dorset UK BH15 2PX

Tel: +44 (0) 1202 674676
Fax: +44 (0) 1202 674776
Email: buzan@buzancentres.com

USA OFFICE

Buzan Centres Inc.
PO Box 4
Palm Beach
Florida
USA 33480

Tel: 001 (561) 881 0188
Fax: 001 (561) 845 3210
Email: buzan@buzancentres.com